To my parents, for teaching me the value of arts and science, to my wife "the amazing Charlo" for being just that, to my children, who despite their protestations otherwise are nowhere misrepresented in this volume, and to my patients, for giving me the greatest honor any man can possibly expect, to trust me with their lives.

-Scott Anderson

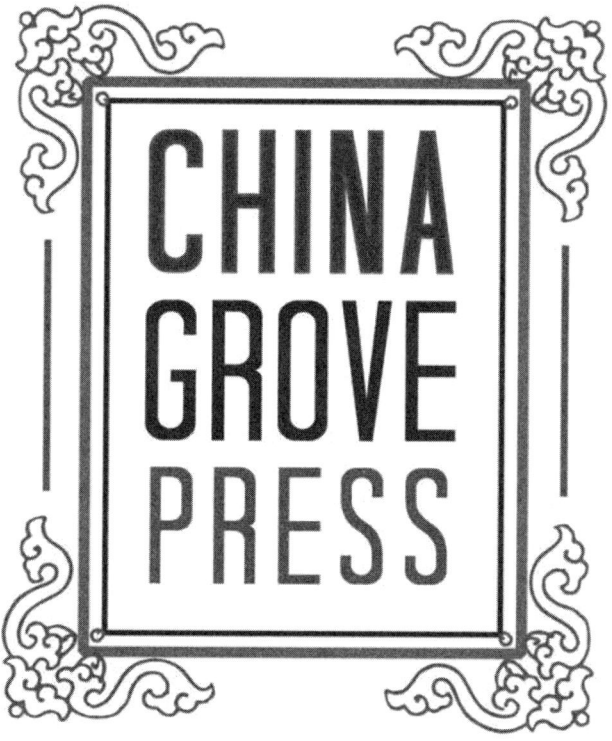

China Grove Press, c/o Magnolia Gazette,
P. O. Box 152, Magnolia, MS 39652,
601-783-2441

Copyright 2012 by R. Scott Anderson M.D.
All rights reserved. No part of this book may be reproduced in any form without the permission of the publisher, except by a reviewer who may quote brief passages.

FIRST EDITION

China Grove Press / IsoLibris Publishing
ISBN 978-0-9852-6710-0

For issues regarding print copies of this book contact www.magnoliagazette.com.
For issues regarding electronic copies of the work contact www.IsoLibris.com.

Original Editors – Karen Evers and Lucius "Luke" Lampton M.D. for the *Journal of the Mississippi State Medical Association*
This volume edited by R. S. Anderson M.D. and Shawnassey Howell Brooks.

TO THE READER:

I suppose some people like to dive right into a book like flinging themselves headlong into a cold stream in early spring. They prefer to let the shock of it wash through their body until they're numbed by it, and then allow the undercurrents to carry them in the downstream direction of the river's own choosing. Not me. I like to stick my toes in gingerly first and test the waters. Life is too short and time is too precious to go swimming merrily but aimlessly with the flow. I want to know something about the who and the why of that stream of consciousness, and most importantly where I'm liable to end up. I want at least a passing acquaintance with the book's author or I'm simply not going anywhere with him.

Thus, I am at loose ends, for my task is to introduce you to this book's creator in a scant few lines. I am in search of just the right words to capture the essence of Dr. Scott Anderson and this scenic and hair raising ride through his life called *The Uncommon Thread*.

There is the Radiation Oncologist, Dr. Anderson, the brilliant, compassionate and beloved healer from Meridian….innovative medical researcher and maverick Mississippi physician leader.

There is Dadosaurus Scotus, the soft-hearted husband of Char and dedicated family man who would drive a thousand miles at warp speed to make it to one of daughter Maddie's horse shows.

There is the unforgettable writer, Russell Scott, who is himself crafted from some strange resilient fabric, a blend of humorist, humanist, philosopher, mystic and madman.

There is the expressive painter, R. S. Anderson, who has not yet plumbed the incredible depths of his artistic talents on canvas. Some of his visual compositions have graced the covers of the **JOURNAL: of the Mississippi State Medical Association**, the publication in which most of these irreverent essays first saw the light of day. When I was dealing with my own cancer experience back in 2008 the physician-artist Scott (my personal long-distance cancer consultant) did a touchingly beautiful oil painting of Jesus and mailed it to me. Inscribed on the back.... "I sent Him to watch over you." He watches over me still from the shelf in my library.

It was during those days of angst and soul-searching that our companion books came to be. Yes, I said 'our' books. The recently released volume, *Una Voce*, has his handprints all over it. Having a book published is a lifelong dream for anyone who writes. My collection would never have seen the light of day if not for the unrelenting efforts and bulldog tenacity of Scott Anderson and our mutual friend Dr. Luke Lampton.

Scott's marvelous impressionistic painting *Voice in the Rain* is the front cover of my meager effort and is the very soul of the book. In fact it was Scott's initial vision to have *Una Voce* be a mixed compilation of both of our **JOURNAL MSMA** scribblings. But, as best laid plans often go, it seemed that our literary sewing styles did not allow the material to mesh seamlessly. Scott's written offerings were cleaved from the original concept book to become this unpredictable crazy quilt collection we call *The Uncommon Thread*.

Let's see... what else can I say about this modern day Renaissance man? Oh, yes, there is the devoted and unflagging friend Scott Anderson who somehow seems to have been blessed with more than 24 hours in each of his days…who answers every phone call and e-mail missive that I toss his way, no matter how trivial its nature. He is doubtless the most multi-faceted, multi-talented, boundlessly energetic person I have ever had the pleasure to know. And he really is a mad genius in the most wonderful kind of way. I always half expect that the next time I see him he will have lopped off one of his ears in a frenzy of creative activity.

So here is the resulting garment you hold in your hand, a vibrant and enduring tapestry woven with love by Dr. Russell Scott Anderson… THE UNCOMMON THREAD.

Dwalia South, MD
March 10, 2012

Contents:

To The Reader -- Dwalia South M.D.

Title	Page
1. The Uncommon Thread	1
2. Lying Mirrors and Other Vexations	4
3. Tuscan Travels	8
4. Stuff That Wears You Out	14
5. Squirrel Story	18
6. Eggs, Beaches, and Shotguns	26
7. A Fleeting Season	29
8. Resolution Revolution	34
9. More and Less	38
10. My Kind of Hunting Story	41
11. The Faith of the Moneychangers	47
12. Heroes	50
13. Chapter Thirteen	53
14. Confabulation Nation	55
15. According to Plan	61
16. Where I Fit in the Food Chain	64
17. Creative Writing	72
18. Teary Sockets	75
19. The One About the Warthogs	81
20. The End of the World	87
21. Caught	94
22. The Ghost and the Book Wright Expansions	99
23. Eavesdropping	112

24. Connect the Dots	116
25. Hard	120
26. Danger-Geenuse At Work	123
27. A Free Man	130
28. Portrait of a Two-Lane Road	133
29. Doc A's Top Ten List on Nutrition	138
30. Canine Behavior	141
31. Tools of the Trade	145
32. Evidence Based	151
33. Loss of Magic	154
34. The Future of Books	157
35. Turtle Rescue Time	159
36. Envy	162
37. Give *Me* Fiction Please	164
38. ZooBots	166
39. Do Not Spill Up Nose!!!	171
40. Boils and Goiters	174
41. Anderson Family Driving School	178
42. Bits of Lint	182
43. Occupy Bourbon Street	184
44. Farewell My Friends	188
About the Author	191

The Uncommon Thread

Hello, and welcome to the funhouse. This collection of stories is the stuff I've been writing for the past couple of years in the JOURNAL: of the Mississippi State Medical Association. Now, why a well-respected monthly scientific medical journal would dedicate their last page to the exploration of literary pretentions and not medical invention is anyone's guess.

Like the victims of any infection, I don't suppose they expected me to take hold. But, I kind of snuck up on them.

It started with me agreeing to fill-in for Dr. Dwalia South for one month. Dr. South had a regular column called *Una Voce,* which means "with one voice". It was designed to represent the common voice of medicine. But, she'd gotten herself elected president of the state medical association, and was going have to switch from *Una Voce* to *The President's Page* for the twelve months she was in that office. So she reluctantly agreed to let me write one column to fill in. She planned to have a variety of contributors fill in on a month-to-month basis and try to keep her column intact for the year she was in office. It didn't work out that way.

One column led to a second and then a third and still no one else was stepping up, so I just kept writing. The more I wrote the more things started to get out of control. This wasn't a novel or a screenplay, where I had to keep track of where it was I was trying to get to in the end. I wasn't trying to get anywhere and I didn't know where the end was. There is a seductive quality to spontaneity and I fell in love with being able to write without set goals, or trying to tell about anything specific.

Una Voce was supposed to be the one voice that represented the practicing physician, but always writing about medicine, and noble callings, and compassion, and all the preconceived crap that doctors are supposed to write about bored me stiff. So I didn't. I wrote about making movies. I wrote about going to Italy and drinking wine. I wrote about hunting. Heck, I even wrote about squirrels. And through it all I wrote about my family and my life.

Poor *Una Voce*, a madman was at the wheel and the columns veered from here to there uncontrollably. They became their own little living things. If I tried to re-write one it would morph and turn into something completely different than whatever it was I originally started out trying to say. Being the creator that was no longer in control was a fun, fun place to be.

I started to think of my little creations as fluid rather than form. I just let them do whatever they wanted for almost a year and when that was over, I was done. I wrote a farewell column, and went back to work on other projects.

But things didn't work out the way I planned either. Dr. South was diagnosed with cancer, and so, as she went through her surgery and the treatment that followed her surgery, *Una Voce* and I careened along. The stories continuing to find their own direction down a jagged and imprecise stream of conscious.

"What in the hell is this?" My left-brain (and sometimes the editor) would demand.

"Don't ask me to explain it," my right-brain would beg, "just read it. Then you'll feel it."

"But what are they supposed to feel?" My left-brain would counter. "Readers want things to relate to one another. They want to know what to expect."

Everybody wants a common thread.

So to make the two sides of my brain knock it off and give me some peace and quiet inside my own head, I tried to come up with an explanation of what it was I wanted to do, and this is what I said:

"What is it about our lives that prepare us to be physicians? Is can't simply be our education, and it had to be there before medicine was our vocation? It happens all around us every day we practice, and I don't think it will stop when we retire. We are what we are because of the millions of tiny incidents in our lives that build up like threads woven into a fabric. That fabric of what we are is what allows us to function as the physicians we can become. It is like taking thread to make a cloth, then taking that cloth

and making a garment.

Medicine we think of as a white coat, but it just looks white because each thread, although it's a different color, shines with promise and adds to the whole.

I want to show it all, the threads, the fabric, all of it. Not just the coat."

Dr. South understood what it was that I was doing while she was gone, probably better than I did, and it was she that came up with the name for my new column and this collection.

See, it isn't the common thread that I wanted to ever show in the first place. It's the uncommon thread, the infinite number of uncommon threads that we weave together to form the fabric of who we are.

Lying Mirrors and Other Vexations

Do you have a mirror? You know, one of those shiny things over the sink in your bathroom that you can see yourself in?

"Sure," you reply, "doesn't everyone?"

I know everybody has one, but I'm growing increasingly concerned with each passing day, that our reliance on things like computers, video links, and special effects is impairing our ability to interpret what it is we see in real life. Alright, hands up; how many of you know how to drive a car with a manual transmission or how to use a slide ruler? Some of you raised your hands, but not many. Those of you who are too young to know what I'm talking about can look them up under "historical curiosities" on your cell phones.

Anyway, getting on with where I was going in the first place, I was out in Los Angeles a few weeks ago and I was struck by the schizophrenic nature of the place when it comes to mirror usage.

There are some people that look like they must spend eight hours a day in front of one, so I was sure that bunch knew how to use them. On the other hand, I had the impression that a lot of the young people I saw out there were totally unaware of the existence of mirrors at all. My son, Jackson, who was out there with me and who used to live there assured me that those same young people probably spent every bit as much time in front of a mirror as the people who actually looked like they did.

Which pretty much proves my theory. If those kids spent all that much time in front of their mirrors and still looked like that when they left the house, they obviously didn't know how the things were supposed to work. I thought, "Well, it's just those crazy kids in California." But that part of my theory didn't last too long.

When I arrived back home, I put my luggage in the trunk, got into my car, and drove out of the airport. I was thankful to be back in the south, where people dressed normally and had normal haircuts.

I don't know if it was just that I had started worrying about people knowing how to use mirrors, or if my time away recalibrated my own sense of normalcy, because the first thing I noticed, at the very first stop light I came to, was the woman in the car in front of me. She had, for some inexplicable reason, chosen to style her hair, so that, her head had the distinct appearance of a pyramid. A few lights later it was a woman with her hair shaped like a helmet. Now I don't think either of these things were an accident. You know what I mean; these weren't the kind of thing that can be caused by a convertible top or an open sunroof. These were styling misadventures, the equivalent of falling over a rock ledge and down a cliff. These two woman had spent a good deal of time in front of a mirror, with curlers, and a blow drier, and brushes, and curling irons and before they knew it they were falling down, down, down into a styling freefall and neither one of them seemed to realize what it was that had happened to them.

This was confusing to say the least. If Jackson was correct, at least the kids in California knew that they were doing something unusual. That started me looking at every car I passed on the street on the way home. In car after car I noticed the strange and unusual things, which people, apparently, simply cannot see about themselves.

You think it doesn't apply to you? Take a look at your prom pictures, maybe Aunt Ellen's wedding. What were you thinking when you put those clothes on? How did you possibly think that peach fuzz mustache made you look like Tom Selleck? Who combed your hair when you went to the prom, your sister's horse?

The entire experience made me start to rethink my own relationship with mirrors. So I went into my closet, closed the door, and looked into the full-length mirror my wife had hidden there years before. (As I don't spend a whole lot of time in my closet with the door shut, I haven't seen it in a while.) I was immediately startled to see that some old fat man had followed me in there. Apparently, he was lost or something, so I turned around to try and offer him some help. But when I turned, I was face to face with my chest of drawers.

Now, admittedly I have been having trouble of late with the cleaners and my wife washing my clothes in hot water, but that fat man standing there couldn't be me, could it? I raised my right hand slowly. The stranger followed my motion with his left. I wiggled my fingers, the stranger responded almost immediately. Crap, I thought, as I put my hand on the strangers bulging waistline.

Well at least I wouldn't be calling my doctor about the shrinkage problem I'd been noticing lately. Not that shrinkage problem. This isn't that kind of a book. I'm talking about my feet.

That's another funny thing. Even though my shoe size has gone up over the last few years, my feet are apparently shrinking. When I was in the Navy I wore a size eight and could see my whole foot. When my baby daughter was born I wore an eight-and-a- half and could see from the laces out easily. Now I wear a size nine and can barely see my toes.

I spent a lot of time thinking about my shrinking feet, trying to come up with some explanation of what was happening to them. I thought perhaps it was all a matter of perspective. Perhaps I was getting taller and my feet only appeared to be shrinking because they were getting farther away from my eyes. I was pretty excited about that idea. I had always known that I was very unlikely to be offered a basketball scholarship or a modeling contract. My height had conspired against me in matters such as this in the past. I had convinced myself that now that I was taller that those issues were behind me and that Calvin Klein should be calling any day. The stupid mirror had ruined that. Feet or no feet, I was rounder but no taller.

The British have a term, seeing through *the mirror of love*. It refers to the inability of a lover to see the flaws of his/or her paramour, because they're blinded by their own feelings. Have you ever heard the old saw, 'You'll never be an alcoholic, if you drink less than your doctor'? We can apply that adage to obesity, stress, smoking, or any other deleterious behavior.

Is the patient who is moderately obese, a moderate smoker, a moderate drinker, really that? Or do we need to take a closer look? Do we as physicians, reflect a true image of what a healthy lifestyle is to our patients? Or do we, like the woman with the triangular head, look at the mirror and say, "Looks good to me."

Personally, I prefer the term moderately obese to the embroidery on the hat I received for my fiftieth birthday. It is the name of a wine I do like a lot, but it refers to the stranger I encountered in my closet, not me. It is another frequently used British term, Fat Bastard. You know, truly, I hate that lying mirror. Maybe I need to get somebody in, to adjust the aspect ratio. Obviously, someone set the stupid thing on widescreen. I'd fix it myself, but I don't have any idea where my wife's put the remote.

Tuscan Travels

-Bilingual Doesn't Mean What You Think

Well, I'm back. What do you mean, you didn't notice I was gone? Of course, you were supposed to notice. Otherwise why would I even bring it up? You were supposed to say something polite, like, "Oh we're so glad you're back." Then I say, "Did you miss me?" Then you say...

Oh forget it. Anyway, I'm back. And let me tell you, I love the USA, I love hamburgers, and I sure do love ice in my Coca-Cola.

Why this sudden burst of Ameriphilia? I, like most Americans, love our country. We know that we do somewhere in the backs of our minds, but we don't spend a lot of time thinking about it from day to day. If you really want to know what it is you love most about it, all it takes is going away from it for a little while and spending some time in some other part of the world.

I happen to be one of those guys that can fall into a hole, and come up with roses in his teeth, and a smile on his face... just before I trip and fall back in the hole, and stab the thorns into the roof of my mouth and my tongue in just the right way to nail my mouth shut. That may be why I tend to be somewhat pessimistic.

When my good friend Adelmo somehow, I don't know how, convinced a bunch of wine distributors and winery owners in Italy, that I represented the taste buds of the typical affluent American wine drinker, and that it would be a good idea for me to accompany him on his annual wine tasting trip, I didn't think much about it. It was never going to work out. It was too good to be true, so why waste time thinking about something that was never going to happen?

Next he managed to convince Charlene of the same thing. I don't think the whole taste buds thing fooled her much. She knows what kind of stuff I eat and drink at home. I think she was swayed more by the fact that Adelmo has been written up more than once in Wine Spectator magazine and is one of the true experts in the US today on the subject of Tuscan wines and maybe I would learn something. The other part, and I can't be really sure that it wasn't the larger part, and while she'll never admit it to my face, I think she also realized that if I was off in Italy, that would be two weeks that she didn't have to put up with me bothering her here at home.

So, that was two steps out of the way, but I still didn't think it would really work out, so I didn't bother doing anything to get ready. A couple of months went by. Then without warning, my airline tickets arrived. Charlene put them on my desk with my passport and a note saying that she had cleared my schedule at work. At this point it appeared, even to me, like I was going to go to Italy.

Oh by the way, did I happen to mention that I don't speak a word of Italian. With just a few weeks until I left, my prospects of learning much more than "the bird is swimming", "the horse is fast and blue" type stuff wasn't very good.

Never one to slack on effort once I have actually put things off until there is virtually no chance of success. I bought three books: Learn Italian in Six Weeks (I'd just have to do three lessons a day to shrink it down to fit the two weeks I had to so it in.), Italian for the Beginner, and an Italian phrasebook and dictionary. Then I enrolled in one of those online Italian courses, and downloaded every podcast on learning Italian that they had on i-tunes onto my i-pod. Even with hard work, I knew I couldn't actually do it, but because I'm neurotic, I had to try. I studied at home, I connected at lunch, and I listened to podcasts in the car.

It wasn't until we arrived in Pisa that I realized, even incrementally, what I was up against. Everyone in Italy talks faster than I can hear. They are like a New York lawyer on a cocaine binge. I on the other hand am saddled with southern ears. It takes a certain cadence for me to get what people are saying, even in English, much less in Italian.

This was going to be a working vacation, so I decided that I was just going to have to get to work. I was damned and determined I was going to learn Italian if it killed me.

Well, I guess I better be a little more specific about the work stuff. It kind of depends on how you define work. If the idea of eating some of the best food in the history of the civilized world and having to taste bottle after bottle of splendid wine seems easy to you, then you have no idea of what a toll such hard living can take. The truth is, that on the first day, between all of the eating and the little bit of drinking I did, I got so worn out by lunchtime that I had to lay down and take a nap. That's one of the nicer traditions in Italy. In fact, I liked it so much that I took a nap after lunch every day from then on, (and tried to when I got home, too, but my nurses had other ideas on that subject.)

This wasn't the easy life of the tourist, oh no, I would be living as part of an Italian household on a hillside, overlooking the bright blue of the Mediterranean. Not a feat for the faint of heart. I will tell you, you have to pace yourself. You have to learn quickly that all of the aunts and cousins that go on and on about…

"Oh, what's wrong with him? He hasn't touched a thing."

"The poor man, he eats like a bird."

… are only being polite.

There is something else that you need to learn very quickly. They put that bucket in the middle of the table at the wine tastings for a reason. That reason being, you may want to <u>walk</u> out of the winery later.

I know, you're thinking, eating, drinking, looking out across the water at the island of Elba isn't going to do much about learning Italian, and you'd be right. I began to watch everything I could on Italian television and made Adelmo translate it for me. I will tell you that we have nothing here in the United States that is remotely like Italian television, they have beautiful scantily clad women in wet shirts dancing on desktops, on the news. I'm not sure exactly how what they were saying had anything to do with the news, but at least it didn't take a whole lot of translation and sure livened up the newscast. I may have believed that the newscasters were reporting that the prime minister had turned into a large type of lunch meat but I could interpret the shape beneath the wet fabric flawlessly.

After the first week I found that I could gain some understanding of what was being said, but as far as two-way communication I was still saddled with a crippling debility. I don't know why, but, even with a phrase book and a good idea in my head of what I wanted to say, there was no way I could get it out of my mouth in a way that any Italians could seem to understand it. So I soldiered on eating, drinking, and speaking in one-word sentences. At least I was beginning to have an idea of what people were saying around me. Well, there was that incident when I mistook the grappa I was given to be acqua minerale. That's one of those things it's hard to recover from without tipping folks off that you have no idea what you're doing.

Another time was when we were on our way to a remote winery, winding our way along a little road that the Italian's built somewhere around 312 B.C., called the Via Apia. We call it the Apian Way. Carlo, Adelmo's cousin was driving, me in the passenger seat, and Adelmo was in the back seat riding in a propane powered Alfa Romeo.

Three large men in a fast car, with Italian license plates, for some reason, must not have looked like a typical group of tourists cruising the wine country, at least not to the Carabinieri.

Now the Carabinieri aren't like a local sheriff we have here in the United States, or even a state trooper. These guys are the Italian Military Police. Not in the way we have military police that are there to police the military. They're a branch of the military, designed to police the people.

Well, here we are driving outside a little village headed into the mountains and we see these three military police. You can imagine how picturesque they were, all dressed up in spiffy black uniforms, with shiny high riding boots standing by the roadside, next to a pretty sharp green and white Alfa sports car with the word Carabinieri painted on the side. Two of them were holding big shiny Beretta sub-machine guns and the one that wasn't was looking real hard at our car. Well, all of a sudden, the observant guy throws up a sign that says ALTO, and Carlo gets on the brakes really hard and stops as quickly as he can.

I can tell some of you are starting to get uneasy for me, aren't you? Well, I still haven't really got a grasp of what's going on yet. These guys haven't got any reason to be concerned about a fat American tourist riding around, tasting wine. Unless you count that run-in I had with a couple of them twenty years ago, down in Sicily, when I was there in the Navy on shore leave. But they couldn't know about that just by looking from the side of the road. Could they? Besides, I jumped out of the hotel window and took off through the bushes, that last time, before they ever got a look at my passport. We didn't have anything to worry about.

When we get stopped the observant guy walks over to the window Carlo's got rolled down by now.

"Blablini blabizini tre umo de Sicilia." He said in a crisp, official voice.

"Oh crap." I thought, and rather than keep my mouth shut and let the people who speak Italian take care of the situation, for some reason, I felt compelled to answer.

"Sono Americano. No have benno a Sicilia in venti ani." I replied mangling both Italian and English in a single sentence.

Since Carlo didn't speak a word of English, and my wooden tongue was apparently garbling the fluent Italian I had just offered, he didn't have any more idea what I was trying to say than the policeman. At that point Adelmo began speaking quickly to both Carlo and the police (the truth is, I don't think he had any idea of what I was trying to say either).

After, what seemed like enough conversation to explain the entire history of the Roman Empire, the policeman growled that he wanted our papers. So, I fished out my nine and a half year old passport, in which I was fifty pounds lighter, fit, and tan. Ready to go on safari. I looked at the picture, and thought, this isn't that good either.

"What's up?" I asked Adelmo.

"The policeman would like you to roll down your window." He answered.

Looking over I saw that the guys with the submachine guns had taken up positions on each side of the car, guns relaxed, but in our direction.

"Hell," I thought. "He shouldn't have any trouble shooting me through the window with that thing."

But, I kept this comment to myself not wanting to upset my companions as I rolled down the window, so no bullets could stray and hit the dashboard or rearview mirror if the machine gun had to be discharged.

"What seems to be the problem?" I asked more directly.

"Well," Adelmo explained, "they have been told to keep a sharp eye out for three very bad men from the south, that are on their way here to cause trouble."

"What kind of bad men?" I asked, kind of relieved now, we weren't bad men.

"Very bad men," he answered.

We were in great shape now, nobody was going to think we were very bad men, a little bad maybe, but we were Americans. We're the good guys. I'd just let 'em know what a good guy I was.

"Nice shoes." I said in my best Italian to the guy outside my window, "I really like those attractive puffy pants." I could tell he didn't want to show it, because he gave me one of those sideways looks and snorted through his nose like there was something stuck in it, but those guys were impressed with how friendly I was being. They got things straightened out and we were on our way in only a little over an hour, and they didn't even have to search us.

Stuff That Wears You Out

There's plenty of stuff to wear you out. The older I get the more worn out I feel. It's like a pair of old shoes, they still may have a lot of miles left in them, but they've had a lot of miles come out of them too.

I almost never get too worn out if I don't care what it is I'm doing. If I go to the National Gallery of Art in Washington D.C. and wander around by myself looking at whatever catches my eye I really start to relax. I can do that all day and come out wonderfully refreshed. But you put me in front of the James McNeil Whistler exhibit with three sixth-grade boys and a football and I come out of there totally exhausted and drenched in sweat in about ten minutes. It comes down to Einstein's explanation of relativity:

"Which seems longer, an hour with a pretty girl, on a minute sitting on a hot stove?"

Or maybe the comedian's response to Einstein:

"Sure we get worn out because of relativity. It's my wife's relativity that wears me out most."

This relativistic view explains one of the things that's always puzzled me. Not my wife's relatives, I just threw that in there. However, what I am thinking about does kind of apply to them, just don't tell 'em I said so. The question I'm referring to is; why do older people drive so slowly? When you think of in terms of relativistic time it makes perfect sense. It's because time itself is moving so much faster for them. The weeks, the months, the years seem to be flying by each one faster than the one before. From their point of view they're burning up the highway. Maybe not on the way to Wal-Mart, but certainly on their way to eternity.

Which brings me back to the main thing that wears us down as doctors? Time, we try to control it and schedule it, but it just won't cooperate. We set out each day just trying to get through the schedule we set for ourselves.

While we're doing that life's busy with a sack of brand new, fresh from the factory, monkey wrenches to toss in there. If you don't believe me, remember the last time you had a jammed packed schedule and you got one of those letters asking you to forward all of a certain patient's medical records to the lawyer who wrote you the letter. Just so he could go through them and make sure everything was up to snuff.

I'm betting that at least a little steam got produced when you read it. Which in itself wasted time, then you had to get the chart, review the chart, to try and find out just what in the world they might be looking for, and then you had to get the chart forwarded. Okay so now you're done with that, you get to resume your schedule, but now you're seeing patients who are mad about being kept waiting. You finally finish and walk back to your office, to find your desk buried under a pile of charts adorned with festive little bits of colored tape stuck to just about every other page to show you where you need to sign. Sound familiar?

So we have to come up with some way to deal with all of this stuff before they find you walking around the halls talking into your stethoscope.

"Houston, we have a problem."

As an expert on these matters, I will tell you that talking into your stethoscope is a perfectly normal thing to do, unless you are doing it with the earpieces of the stethoscope in your ears. Then you're talking to yourself, and we all know what that means, and no you cannot bill a separate consultation fee. Very bad form unless you're fond of federal prison.

When you add the socio-political issues to the fact that the verschmicken diseases won't read the textbooks, and have a tendency to do all kinds of things that they're not suppose to do and hardly ever want to respond to treatment the way you want them to. Then what we end up with is something called professional stress.

I don't think this is one of those terms that is all that clear, so I'll try to explain it a little. The stress we're talking about isn't somehow better than some other stress referred to as amateur stress. Nor is it a stress that has somehow taken an advanced degree. It is the stress we have as medical professionals.

If somebody has the audacity to ask you if you feel stressed, do not grab them by the lapels and shake them while shouting.

"Stress, stress…are you talking to me about stress?"

As that tends to make the asker kind of nervous, and can result in people thinking that maybe, just possibly, you may be wrapped just a little bit too tight, or that you are, God forbid, a disruptive physician. Maybe you're suffering from the new malady of "physician burn out".

Stress, in and of itself, is not a bad thing, it strengthens us, and we just have to find ways to deal with it. Being stressed out, on the other hand, is a problem. It erodes our well being, and keeps us from enjoying life.

As physicians we're stressed. We're asked to play on an ever-changing field of scientific, political, legal, and social constraints. Sometimes it seems like as soon as you get out your basketball to head over to the tennis courts and toss the old horsehide around, you get tackled by a lawyer in a referee's uniform that then begins to beat you with a hockey stick, and scream that you fouled him because your foot was past the line when you jumped.

Now stop shaking your heads, and muttering, "What is this idiot talking about now?" Yes, I can hear it all the way down here in Meridian.

I'm talking about identity. We fight and try for years in order to become Dr. So-and-so. It becomes who we are. If you don't believe me, see if the hairs on your neck don't prickle up, just a bit, the next time one of your kid's friends calls you Mr. So-and-so.

What wears us down is the fact that it's hard, sometimes, to take that white coat with Dr. Joe So-and-so MD off. It stops being the symbol of our profession, and begins to be the symbol of who we are, or who we see ourselves as. When that happens, that white coat begins to take on all the attributes of a straight jacket, which keeps us from ever getting out of Dr. So-and-so's world.

I remember reading a few years ago that physicians bought expensive toys like boats, and exotic cars, not for the leisure time and relaxation that these things provide, but for the idea of that relaxation. I bought some race cars a few years ago with the idea that I was going to race them in vintage racing events, I began to tear them apart, to get them ready, so they could be competitive. Most of you know where this is going. No, I didn't get a stable of trophy winning race cars, I got four cars that didn't run and boxes and boxes of new parts and tools, that I haven't touched, because I'm too busy to be hauling race cars all over the place, and I'm too busy to spend all the hours necessary to get the cars back together. But I still keep them, and not because I'm pig-headed, like my wife accuses, but because I might have enough time soon. I just don't know when soon is.

The point is, Dr So-and-so has it tough, he's in a swirling kaleidoscope that'll only speed up its ever-changing patterns as the years pass, and he'll continue to get more burned up, and more burned out all the time, if he doesn't get a break. He'll continue to be driven, committed, frustrated, confused, and then driven to overcome that confusion. He does it because he's a physician, and he's been taught all of his life that physicians are special.

The trick is, we don't always have to be special. There's nothing wrong with being "plain old Joe" some of the time. That's who we were before we put these white coats on. That, in fact, is our refuge, and that's where Tom Petty and Stevie Nicks are wrong, sometimes you do have to live like a refugee.

So, if you see me driving an old car without a windshield, or sitting in a golf cart with my daughter, having a make believe tea party, don't think, "Oh gosh, what's going on here? Dr. Anderson has lost his mind." It's just me, Scott, and that's okay.

Squirrel Story

My sum total of wisdom from raising seven children is this; there's no use threatening to call child-protective services, to come and take them away. They won't believe you (the kids, not the child protection people). Three of my children just ran into the den, jumped around in front of the television and informed me that I'm now the grandfather of a baby squirrel that the dog that they adopted after finding it on a roadside drug in. Maddie, who is nine-years-old, and Charlene, who is forty-something years-old, going on nine, managed to rescue the tiny thing from the dog's mouth, inflicting only minimally more damage than the dog was by chewing on it.

"We're going to feed it with a bottle." Maddie announced.

"Who is?" I asked. I should have known better, but I just wanted to be sure nobody was under the impression that I was going to be the one feeding it.

"I am." She said.

Thank goodness, we already have a parrot, some other bird, three dogs, and I think three horses. The last thing I want is something else to feed. That's how they're so sure I'm not going to call child-protective services. They know I'm never going to take care of all of these animals by myself.

Then it came. "NO. I am." This started the inevitable sequence of:

"I am."

"NO. I am."

"I am."

"NO. I am."

Repeat until intolerable, with each child doubling their volume with each repetition until they're all screaming their brains out and you have to holler even louder just to be heard.

"Knock it off, or I'm cooking the stupid thing and eating it." I shouted.

King Solomon used the same tactic on those two women that wanted the same baby. It worked like a charm for him.

"You are not cooking Lilly"

"Mommy, Daddy's hollering at us for no reason."

"She's not stupid."

All came back at once so that it was impossible to decipher which response came from whom.

"Who's Lilly?" I asked.

"The squirrel!" They all shouted in unison.

"Momma says you have to check her out to be sure she's okay." The child we all refer to as "Miss Bossypants" announced officially, hands on her hips, chin stuck out.

"Alright, bring her in here then, and I'll see if she's tender enough to eat." I answered. I really don't know why I do these things. It's meant to torture them, but invariably it ends up only driving <u>me</u> crazy. It's kind of like the old stories about why you shouldn't wrestle a pig in mud…you both get dirty, and the pig likes it. By the time they get through screaming for Charlene, and giving me lectures on why we don't eat our pets, I'm convinced that I would have been far wiser just to have just kept my big mouth shut. King Solomon must have only used that stuff on adults because it doesn't work worth beans on screaming children.

So they brought me the squirrel, still covered with drool, with a few scratches on her flanks, but otherwise intact.

"She looks okay, but we'll have to see how she's doing in the morning." I said.

This isn't my first injured squirrel. In fact, there isn't a kid in the house that hasn't been through this before. Even Maddie knows the proper recipe for squirrel formula. We are, at this point, I suppose, a semi-professional squirrel rescue facility. (We're probably going to go pro next year, that's where the big bucks are.) Every time there's a hurricane or a bad storm in the autumn we end up with a new batch of baby squirrels. Sometimes, we find them, sometimes the dogs do, and sometimes we get them from the neighbors or our vet.

My advice, to any of you considering climbing up a tree and seeing if you can't liberate a baby squirrel of your own, is: FORGET IT, especially if you have children. Don't get me wrong, they're very cute and sweet as babies, but they grow up (the squirrels, not the children, well maybe both of them.) They start biting as they mature, particularly if they're males or you have more than one of them (the squirrels are what I was referring to again, however, this statement also is equally true of children. This is getting too confusing. For the sake of convenience, I will only be talking about squirrels from this point on. Unless, I specifically say I am talking about children.) I don't know why the squirrels decide to start biting. Maybe they talk about it and reason, "Hey if we bite them every time they try to pick us up, perhaps, they'll let us go." Or, maybe they prefer to be with each other rather than being picked up by some giant hand that's no longer trying to feed them a bottle. Anyway, whatever the reason, eventually, you have to release them. There's the problem. First you have to convince the children that setting them free is for the squirrels own good, and not just because they stink, bite you, and if they get out take about an hour to get back into the stupid cage. The first time we went through this Maddie was only five or six. The release phase started with a serious discussion with all of the children, about the need to begin to get the little nippers (literally) ready for their arboreal paradise. That's how we told the children they felt, for them, trees were like heaven.

For the most part, I was afraid that we were just feeding the hawks, and if Maddie saw one of her little pals flying along clenched in the talons of a bird of prey, I wanted her to think that the little guy had just sprouted wings and flown off to his squirrely maker. Maddie is so tender hearted that she adopted a poor baby snapping turtle for a good part of that summer, unfortunately, it escaped after a few months when I took it with me to teach it how to go fishing.

They didn't buy it, so, when reason failed, I was forced by necessity to try the old guilt strategy. You know, every parent has had to use it for something. It goes something like this:

You: "You know Daddy's getting older?"

Child: "Are you really older than dirt?"

You: "Who said I was older than dirt?"

Child: "Mommy."

You: "Well never mind about dirt. You don't want Daddy to have a heart attack or a stroke or something, do you?"

Child: "Why would you have a heart attack?"

You: "The squirrels are trying to give me one."

Child: "The squirrels aren't trying to give you one."

You: "Yes they are."

Child: "How?"

You: "Every time they bite me or make me run around the house after them, they make my blood pressure go up. You know what happens when people's blood pressure goes up?

Child: "No what."

You: "They can have a heart attack or stroke."

Child: "Is that why your face turns all red and you start hollering cuss words?"

You: "Yep, those are the first signs of a heart attack or stroke."

Child: "Should we get rid of Dylan?"

You: "That's ridiculous, why would we get rid of your brother?"

Child: "Because he almost makes you have a stroke every time he does something bad, like when he wrecked the car."

You: "We're not getting rid of your brother!'

Child: "He's a lot more trouble than the squirrels."

Anyway, you get the idea. When that didn't work I told them that I thought that it was time for the squirrels to have climbing lessons. Allison, my older daughter commented that she didn't think that I was the one to be giving the squirrels climbing lessons because my toenails were nowhere near sharp or strong enough to support my weight on the side of a tree.

So, after Char took the kids to school, we decided to take the oldest, and worst behaved of the lot (of squirrels) outside for some climbing practice in a pear tree that was about eight feet tall. When I sat the little guy down at the base of the tree, he took off and ran straight under Dylan's truck, who was also trying to get ready to go to school. I must admit, it was rather amusing to watch Dylan chasing a squirrel from wheel to wheel for ten or fifteen minutes, but then Char said he was going to be late for school, so she made me help him. So we got the squirrel between us. He was pretty much trapped, or so I thought. He ran straight between my legs. When I grabbed for him, he took one bounce off my thigh and darted through the chain-link fence and was into the woods and then thirty feet up a tree before I finally lost sight of him. I may have been slightly less than polite when

Char asked if I was just going to leave him out there. She later accused me of saying that I didn't give a damn what she did with the stupid little tree rats, but I'm sure that I remember offering to work with the two remaining squirrels after work.

I finally got to work, late, and spent a good part of the day trying to catch up, and had just about done so by 3:00 when the receptionist called to tell me my wife was on the line. When I put the phone to my ear, it sounded as if an air raid siren was going off.

"Do you hear that?" Charlene demanded.

"What, do you think I'm deaf? What is that? Where are you?" I asked.

"I'm in the back yard and that's your daughter," she said, silently inferring that I was a bad father for not knowing as much.

"What, did you do, run over her with the car?" I asked trying to figure out what was happening.

"No, this is all your fault."

"MY FAULT? I'm still at work."

"You said to let the other two squirrels go, so that's what I did."

"Well, then tell her how happy they are up in the trees." I answered, trying to keep the party line.

"That's what I was doing. We were looking up at little Addy up there holding onto the tree trunk, and I was telling Maddie how much she loved having the breeze blowing around her and how happy she was, when she let go."

"What do you mean, let go?" I asked.

"Let go of the tree," she said, her voice rising, "she let go of the tree and just fell right at Maddie's feet."

"Is she OK?" I asked.

"Does she sound like she's OK?"

"Not Maddie, the squirrel?" I tried to clarify.

"The squirrel is DEAD." She shouted. Then more softly, she added, "I tried to give her CPR."

"For crying out loud, how far did she fall?"

"All the way to the ground, you idiot."

"That wasn't what I meant…" I started.

"Just get home. Now." She demanded.

"Baby, I still have two patients that are coming in later. The squirrel's already dead. There's not much I can do about that." I tried to explain.

"You have to get the other one, he's still up there." She said, clearly exasperated that I was so slow. "Do you hear your daughter?"

Over the line I could hear Maddie sobbing, "Hold on Ivan, daddy's coming to get you."

"Alright, alright I'll be right there."

When I arrived, Maddie and Char were standing at the foot of the largest pine tree in a yard full of big pine trees, and yes, there was the unfortunate Ivan, clinging to the trunk…sixty feet up. Char knowing that I would be pushed for time had already gotten the extension ladder…a twenty foot extension ladder.

"This isn't going to reach." I explained.

"I couldn't set it up…please, just try…"

So I set up the extension ladder climbed all the way up, and was still about thirty-five feet short. As I got down, knees shaking only slightly, and turned around, she was holding the pool skimmer, which she had extended to its full fourteen feet.

"Just try this…"

So, now I was back up the ladder, knees now really shaking, and arms shaking as well, as I tried to hang on to the tree with one arm and swing the skimmer wildly with the other, still twenty feet below the terrified squirrel.

"Be careful… you're waving it too hard, Try to stay in control…Now just see if you can get it a little higher." Char offered.

At this point, two things happened simultaneously. Our neighbor Mary pulled up with her two children to say hi, and I exploded in a fit of gloriously colorful profanity, that stood up to anything I had ever heard from a master chief petty officer during my days in the Navy. I was so engrossed in finding the exact phrases to describe the stupidity of standing on the top rung of a twenty foot ladder, clinging to a tree, and swinging a fourteen foot pole with a net on it, that I never noticed her arrival.

"Mary and her kids are here!!!" came up from below me, sharply.

"Hi guys," I said, pretending nothing had happened.

"Well, I guess we'd better be going," Mary replied diplomatically, despite a reddened face. "Good luck with the squirrel."

"Maybe if I back the truck up…" Char shouted up at me, as Mary's SUV pulled out the back driveway.

"Are you out of your mind?" I replied, as politely as possible.

"Well what are we going to do? We have to do something."

"I have a plan," I said as I climbed down, "you and Maddie go in the house and get a shoe box for Addie and I'll take care of Ivan."

"What are you going to do?" Maddie asked. Charlene knew better.

"I have a great plan, I'm going to try and get him to come down and get some food." I answered, thinking quickly.

"But he can't climb down." She replied.

"He just doesn't know he can climb down. When he starts thinking about the food, he'll forget he can't climb down." I said, just as if it made sense.

"Oh. Ok," she said, and holding Charlene's hand went into the house.

She'll hear a shotgun I thought, as Dylan drove up. Then I knew what it was we had to do.

"Hey Dyl, Come here. Grab a can of tennis balls."

So we started, him with a strong arm, throwing the tennis balls at the tree, over the squirrel making it inch backward down the tree. When we had him about half-way down, the back door slammed signaling Maddie and Charlene's return, Dylan's throw went low, almost hitting the squirrel's tail and as everyone watched Ivan ran up the tree into the branches, jumped to another tree and was gone.

"See," Maddie said, "all he needed was some climbing lessons."

For the next two years we saw Ivan almost every day, sometimes it was hard for me to distinguish him from any of the other innumerable grey squirrels around our house, but somehow, Maddie always knew.

Update: Ever since a much shorter version of this story first appeared in Una Voce, I've been asked, "So, what happened to Lilly?" The short answer is she's fine.

She's the first squirrel that has remained semi-domesticated. She's been set free but stays near the house. She's built her own nest high up in a tree and stays in it during the day but chooses to return every night to sleep in a large cage with a small door at the base of her tree in a gated courtyard.

She finds her own acorns, but will climb down her tree any time

Maddie or Charlene call her. She's happy to run up their arms to sit on their shoulders and beg for cashews.

Many times, as I drink my coffee in the morning, she'll appear on the windowsill and tap on the glass for me to put some nuts out. She won't allow me to touch her, but comes back and eats her nuts as soon as I shut the window.

I think she would be even friendlier with the girls, but they don't encourage it, they're afraid of predators. Several times I've looked out into the yard to see Maddie, broom in hand, locked in fierce combat with the neighbor's tomcat. Lilly watching from a branch high above the action. I think she's gonna do just fine.

Eggs, Beaches, and Shotguns

What do all of these things have in common? That's the kinds of riddles we grew up with in our house. With four kids separated by six years, we were always trying to come up with something to show which one of us was the smartest. If one of us heard a riddle in school or church, we'd drag it home, acting as if we were the ones that had thought of it our own self, and during dinner toss it out. If someone came up with the right answer, we'd be crestfallen. Immediately replying, "That was an easy one, wasn't it?" to save face. If a bunch of wrong answers were offered up, the asker would begin to give out clues. Tossing out crumbs of wisdom to the obviously mentally inferior siblings. When the answer was finally revealed, somebody, never me mind you, would say, "Yeah, I thought of that, but I didn't want to say it."

Things aren't really all that different in the adult world, sometimes connections are easy to figure out, like the words in the title (they all have shells), other times they're tougher. Sometimes we don't make the connections ourselves, and have to get them explained to us.

Some of you may remember my big idea, to write an open letter to our patients, called *Saving Lives*:

"A letter from physicians to the citizens of the United States...our friends...our patients. —Written in the way you would write to a dear friend who wasn't a health care professional, in a voice anyone can understand. —Written to shed light, not generate heat. —To show the concerns of our hearts, not manipulate. Written by a group, not by an individual, so that the ring of truth is undeniable and can't be discredited by personal attacks."

When I envisioned it, I hoped to have contributions from a hundred or so physicians in our state. I wrote that invitation and sat back waiting for the offers to pour in. The response surprised even me...only one.

At first I was incredulous. Maybe, I'd written down the wrong e-mail address. Maybe everyone lost it before they got a chance to read it. A thousand reasons bounced around my head, but none of them made much sense.

While I was still worrying about this unexpected turn of events, I attended a fundraiser for one of the Lieutenant Governor candidates, the one that wasn't a trial lawyer. After several individuals made comments on how important the Lieutenant Governor was to the introduction and progress of legislation, our attention was directed to the optimistically large jar labeled, "campaign contributions". A lot of the people there were physicians, so I thought, "Well we're good." Once again I found myself amazed, this time at the small amount of cash collected. We came up way short of our anticipated goal.

An attorney, who had organized the event, said something that took some thinking. She said, "Physicians are without a doubt the most powerful political force in this state, and probably in our country. You just can't convince them of that. They're too busy helping their patients, to really help their patients."

It took me a minute to let that one sink in...We're too busy helping our patients to really help our patients. That doesn't even make sense...this is another one of those stupid riddles, but the more I thought about it the truer it sounded, and the more it explained both of the things that were puzzling me.

We're battered daily by the importance of the ceaseless minutiae of medicine, sodiums, potassiums, ruptured viscera, fractures, and infections take all of our energies, and when we get done with them...well, we never get done with them. How can stupid laws and politics and stuff like that, that we've never even been trained in, be just as important as the medical decisions we make? They are, and in fact, they will exert an even greater influence on the overall health of the population we serve, than any of our individual efforts, and their effects will be longer lasting.

Saving Lives is dead, it was a good idea, but unfortunately quite naïve.

Se la vies, or se la guerre, take your pick, but pick you must, because both life and the battles we face as part of it, require us to pick. To become a part of the battle takes effort, it takes a sense of urgency and necessity. It takes the romantic assurance to be unafraid to look like Don Quixote.

"Wait a minute," I can hear you saying, "This guy is quitting on his project, and he gets on his high horse and starts lecturing us about commitment and trying to realize our political power. Aren't these kind of contradictory messages?"

The high horse that was, at the same time, the don's mighty charger and nothing but a spavined plow horse to the rest of the world gives us a clue. These too, are contradictory images, but Rocinante means reversal. Sure, I'm a romantic, but I'm not an idiot. Its okay to ride full tilt, lance drawn, at a windmill, if you really believe it's a dragon. It's lunacy to do it, once you realize it's a windmill…well, wait a minute, even if it is a windmill, it still might need some attacking. We just need the right weapon…Sancho, we got a bazooka?... What do you mean, we should write something smaller?... How can that be better than a bazooka?...All right then, anyway, I already thought of that, I just didn't want to say it…Why?...Well, because it sounded too simple., and besides, ever since I got my first set of those green plastic Army men, I always did want to shoot a bazooka.

A Fleeting Season

I know scientifically that time is a constant. A second, a minute, an hour, and a day remain the same in every month and in every season of the year. By all rights then, they should all be <u>perceived</u> as constant throughout the year, but they aren't. February is shortest month of every year, whether it's a leap year or not, but when you're waiting for the winter to end and the spring to finally spring out from under a layer of snow, it seems to drag on forever. It isn't quite as bad here in the south, but the further north you go the longer February gets.

If you don't believe me ask my sister. She and her family live in Alaska. They get so depressed by the winter that they have to buy sunlamps and lay under them for thirty or forty minutes a day to keep from losing their minds. Well maybe that's a little drastic. Okay, so their mental health might not be quite that precariously balanced, but for some reason laying under the sun lamps makes them all feel better.

There are some people that think that it is because the nights get so much longer than the days that it makes you depressed, to some extent, and that depression is what makes it seem like time refuses to move at the same pace that it does all the rest of the year. This isn't simply a psychological depression. It may actually be an endocrine mediated metabolic slow down as a result of a hormone called melatonin.

There is a month though that defies temporal description, December. As a child, waiting for Christmas, December was at least three months long. But, now that I'm older, December has become the shortest month of the ever-shortening years. Everything is going along at the right pace, football season starts, then its Halloween, and in a little while Thanksgiving comes along, then whoosh, time warps.

It's as if the year funnels down, and everything is being compressed as tightly as possible to get everything in before the year ends. If you've ever watched as a coin goes around and around faster and faster as it travels down a funneled cone, until it simply drops away. That's how this time of year feels to me.

It usually starts with the shopping. Then the parties, receptions, dinners, and all of the other social commitments start to get more and more frequent, until you have more parties than days. The pressure to shop increases as you have less and less time before the big day and you still don't even know who all you need to buy stuff for.

Then BAM it's Christmas. Parents with too little sleep are awakened to the sound of anxious children, who have been threatened with death if they go into the living room until everyone's ready. Moms photograph, videotape, make breakfast, and try to get everything cleared away so they can get a start on making Christmas dinner. Dads gather the boxes and wrapping paper together in a giant pile. Try to find out where those diabolical elves have hidden the battery compartments and then fight to get the five million restraining wires holding all of the toys in the boxes off, so the kids can play with them.

When we get through all of that, we rush around trying to see all of the family members we can and call all of those we can't. Then we eat a gigantic Christmas dinner, fight to stay awake while we clean every piece of china in the house, because for some reason we needed every piece we had to eat a meal six times bigger than we eat any other day of the year except Thanksgiving. Finally we fall into an exhausted slumber wondering where the holiday went.

With all of the hustle and bustle we miss a lot in those fleeting December days. Of course, the kids won't miss the obviously inebriated, yellowish nicotine stained Santa looking at rifles in the sporting goods store. Especially when he announces the obvious, in a sloshy roar.

"Kids always get a little nervous when they see old Santa packing heat."

The tragedy is that we miss the small, beautifully poignant moments that are happening all around us. So, I wanted to take this time, when we're all rushing around trying to get ready for Christmas, to share something that happened to me way back in another century, at the dawn of civilization, when I was still a resident.

My attending at the time was a wee Scottish woman, with an intellect as bright and penetrating as a lighthouse beacon. She didn't always hold the same opinion of me, evidenced by her tendency to refer to me, on occasion, as "you blockhead." This usually occurred when I would happen to forget that some organ or tumor I was having trouble defining on an x-ray had already been removed surgically. Keep in mind, this was back at the dawn of post-operative radiotherapy. Shut up! I know it's a flimsy excuse! Anyway, stop sniggering, so I can go back to the story. She and I had drawn Christmas Day call, and, of course, we got called. The holiday protocol was for the resident to go in, gather up the important details, do the history and physical and then call the attending to discuss their findings.

I arrived in the ER to find that the patient we'd been called about was an old friend named Ellen. I had treated Ellen for her lung cancer earlier in the year. When I asked her what was wrong I watched as Ellen's face contorted. She would start to speak then stop, start and stop.

"I…I…I…t t t t talk. I…I…I…" she struggled valiantly.

"Just take your time." I said sitting in the chair beside her and leaning forward.

"C c c c cannnn't t t t t t talk." Ellen fought on, her frustration growing.

The condition is called aphasia. She knew what it was that she wanted to say. She just couldn't catch the words she needed to say what it was that she needed to say and then string them together to say anything. This was new. She had been articulate and in good spirits the last time I'd seen her.

"Just rest a minute, and I'm going to have them give you some medicine in your IV that will help." I said.

Aphasia, I wrote on the line that was labeled Chief Complaint and wrote an order for the IV steroids to stop the swelling around the tumors I was already fairly sure what I was going to find.

"I'll be back in a few minutes," I said. "I'm going to go and look at the CT scan of your head."

Even without contrast the tumors growing in Ellen's brain were easy to see, scattered throughout her cortices like a hundred tiny Christmas ornaments. This many lesions having spread to her brain from her lungs meant that she had a fifty percent chance of surviving in six weeks if we didn't treat her and only about the same chance of surviving six months if we did.

Our brains come with a whole lot of things that are supposed to protect them and in this case most of them were working against us. Our brains are inside a hard bony case, our skulls, that's there to keep us from getting a concussion every time we bump our head. This is generally a good thing, unless there's something extra trying to grow in there. There's no room for extra stuff. Think of your skull as a metal lunchbox full of sandwiches (your brains are the sandwiches) the whole lunchbox is full of sandwiches. Now if you throw an apple into the lunchbox and slam the lid, what is going to get mashed? The apple or the sandwiches? Our brains are soft like the sandwiches and the tumors are hard and firm like the apple. I think you get the picture.

The second thing is a thing called the blood-brain barrier. Our brains have a layer of lipid or fat that keep poisons, like chemotherapy from getting into the brain. Keeping poisons away from our brain is so important because we have all of the brain cells we're ever going to get when we're born. Any of them that get destroyed aren't coming back, so our body is designed to protect them.

Time was of the essence, we would have to start the treatments as soon as possible, because the tumor was growing, and by growing was destroying irreplaceable brain cells.

We needed the radiation to do two things, kill the tumors, or at least keep them from growing, and open up the blood-brain barrier so chemotherapy would have a chance of being effective.

I explained all of these things to Ellen. She shook her head to show me that she understood as I spoke. I called my attending, who I'm now allowed to call Beth, and told her that we were going to have to treat Ellen tonight, then relayed the details of the case. Patient presented with expressive aphasia after falling at home. CT scan shows multi-focal bilateral brain metastases with several having significant swelling. She said she'd be there in thirty minutes.

This was back in the days when the physicians could still run the machines, do the calculations, treat the patient, and then wheel them back to their room without help. It took time for Beth to get there, more time to do the set up, and more time for me to do the calculations and Beth to check them. When we finally got ready to treat her, Ellen was so worn out she sat slumped in a wheelchair with her head in her hands.

"I'm sorry." I said, "This has to be a terrible Christmas."

"No," She answered, "This has to be a wonderful Christmas."

It's the aphasia I thought to myself. Because, she couldn't think of the words she wanted, she was just echoing back what I had just said. But what she said next showed a clarity of thought, I still rarely possess.

"It's the last Christmas I'm ever going to have," she said determinedly, looking up from the wheelchair. "It <u>has</u> to be a wonderful Christmas."

Later, with the patient returned to her room, I walked out of the back door of our department with Beth, and wished her a Merry Christmas, anxious to get home to my two sons.

"I hope you realize the gift you were given tonight," she replied.

I must have looked somewhat confused. My mind slowed by a sadness that swirled around in my heart like the snow in the parking lot.

Looking me in the eye, she explained. "Before I can make you a good oncologist, I need to make you a better human. So you can get past the facts of the case, and be able to see the person in front of you. What you just saw, what you just heard, remember it, it may not make you a better doctor, but it will make you a better person."

I still struggle with the responsibility of that lesson.

Resolution Revolution

Happy New Year! It seems like I've been waiting to say that since mid-October. About then I start feeling kind of cramped, it's almost like there aren't enough days left in the year to really get comfortable any more. Anything you try to do, or any plans you make seem to come crashing up against Thanksgiving or Christmas somehow. Besides I always hate waiting until the last minute to do anything, and no that doesn't prove I'm obsessive-compulsive, I don't care what my wife says.

So come on in, have a seat, and make yourself at home. There's plenty of room. We've got 365 days in front of us. You can go ahead and stretch out. No squeezing things in at the last minute here, it's clear sailing right up until Easter.

Have you got all of your resolutions made already? In place, ironed out, and ready to go? Well, I wish you luck with them. It's always good to start the New Year with good intentions. Forget all of that stuff about the road to hell being paved with the worthless little monsters. I'm sure you're going to do better this year than you've done in the past. Well, I'm not really. I was just saying that to be polite.

Have I made any? Well, I've never really had much success with them in the past myself so you might say I'm pessimistic on the subject. But, to make it easy to keep track of I just rewrite the same list every year, year in and year out I stick with the same little list. I like to keep things manageable, so I limit myself to just five. I know it would be more of a challenge if I tried to switch it up some. I might even have a better chance of being successful keeping a few of them, but I'm a creature of habit and I've always felt it was best to try and stick with what I know.

That way, I never have that much to feel guilty about either. Year after year the outcome is pretty predictable. I have a decade's worth of past failures to base my expectations on.

So what are they? Most years, the top spot on the list has been to quit cussing. Unfortunately, most years it's also the first resolution to get broken. It's not my fault. Everyone knows it's impossible to watch all the bowl games that are on TV on New Years Day without some blind referee blowing a call in an important game…and you can guess the rest.

A relative to that one is the old bad temper resolution. I may seem calm and collected at all times, but once in a while I have been known to…anyway I usually resolve to try and quit losing my temper so much. I usually just tie the first three resolutions all together because breaking one usually leads to breaking at least two at the same time. That third one has been to try to get myself to church more. You can see how these three are related. I thought that going to church would make me less likely to lose my religion, as the old timers say. Thus, saving both of the first two resolutions at the same time.

The big triumvirate was usually followed by a vow to make an effort to spend more time with my family. Every time I've made this resolution in the past Charlene, my wife, has found it necessary to impose a bunch of ridiculous constraints on this poor resolution. She always insists that time in front of a TV or in a deer stand doesn't count as "quality" time with the family. Don't ask me why, what could help you bond with your eight-year-old daughter more than watching the Sugar Bowl or the Final Four?

Last but not least, there's the biggie, the biggest of the big, to lose weight and get more exercise. Hell, (there goes number one) I should be an expert on that one by now. The way I figure it, in my adult life, so far, I've lost about six hundred pounds, and I'm still fifty pounds ahead. Now that's a good trick if you're talking about the British monetary system, but in terms of body mass it's not much of an accomplishment.

Well this year I'm doing something different. I'm staging a revolution, right here on this printed page, I've decided that I'm not making a bunch, well I guess five isn't all that big of a bunch, but I'm not making any resolutions.

It's not that I think that I don't need any improvement. I just don't believe any of those things is going to make me any better of a person, and I'll tell you why…

Now that I'm a published author, that makes me an artiste`, and everybody knows that artiste's don't cuss, they use language creatively. I think I even took a course on that back in college. So that ones done. No, no going back for me. Now that my cussin' is an integral part of my creativity it's gotta stay.

Losing my temper, well that's just a part of my artistic temperament, and who knows what could happen if we mess with that.

As far as spending more time with my family, after raising seven kids, I've spent so much time with my family I'm about bald from pulling my hair out, and with two twelve year-olds and an eight year-old still at home, my life has started to feel like a Bill Cosby routine. Besides, after Holton told Charlene about all the creative new words he learned after we spent a week in the wilderness with the Boy Scouts (and I will say we were only lost half the time, the other half of the time we knew the canoe was going in the wrong direction, there just wasn't anything we could do about it) she suggested I might want to cut back on some of those types of activities, so that one's out too.

The church thing is probably still not a bad resolution, but I'm already a white, heterosexual, Christian, adult male, and Lord knows we're already responsible for about everything that's wrong with the world today as it is. If you don't believe me, ask anybody you see on CNN or Fox protesting about just about anything, and they'll let you know real fast. It's all our fault. Since I'm not going to make any special effort to be any more white, heterosexual, adult or male, and I wouldn't know how to, if I wanted to. I don't guess I better try to be any more Christian either. I'll just upset more people and make them drive up to Washington and march around holding signs and all.

That still leaves exercise and weight loss. Well, who wants to mess with one measly resolution? Besides, there've been a lot of new ideas on all that.

I read an article this year that shed a whole new light on all that exercise stuff. It turns out, it's not all it's been talked up to be. In fact, people who ran even one marathon had a life expectancy seven years shorter than the average slug, who walked everywhere and slurped down hamburgers and French fries by the sack full. Well, maybe that wasn't exactly what it said, but that was the general idea.

I also found a new favorite book this year, *Rethinking Thin*, in which the author makes the wonderful point that, in looking at statistics since the civil war, that the average American today is four inches taller than were their kin at the time of that unfortunate venture. Her idea is that because we are freer of disease and adequately nourished, that we are finally able to realize out genetic potential for height. So, we should apply that same logic to weight, we're not fatter, we're just better realizing our genetic potential for mass. We need to get in touch with the governor and legislature fast on this one. Mississippi is not fiftieth in the country on obesity, no siree, we are first in the country in helping our population in reaching their maximum genetic potential for something. What could possibly be wrong with that? We should all be jumping around and holding up our finger, like they do at football games and hollering, "We're number one, we're number one..." instead of moping around hanging our heads because we're too fat. We aren't fat, we're massive. MASS...IVE, MASS...IVE, MASS...IVE. GO INERTIA GO.

Are y'all buying this? Let me know as soon as you can, because I thought I'd run it past you, before I tried it on Charlene. I used to think she was kind of slow sometimes, but I'm beginning to suspect that she's deliberately missing the brilliance of my logical arguments for the things I do.

Well, welcome to the year of the resolution revolution. Revolution is usually a good thing, unless you're French, or Russian, or live in a third world country, or are married to a woman like Charlene, who's gonna point all those other ones out as bad ideas too.

More and Less

Let me let you in on one of the basic facts of life, and no, you don't have to be a doctor to know this one, everybody wants more!

"More what?"

Who knows? More money for some, more fulfillment for others, or perhaps just more love, a lot of times it varies. It may be one thing one day and another thing the next. What we want more of is variable. The feeling that we need more of something is universal. For me what I need more of depends on the season and what mood I'm in. In the fall I need more jackets. In the spring I feel like I have a shortage of golf clubs. Never mind that I have closets overflowing with both and I have more of either than I can ever reasonably use. I don't have the one I need now.

And I'm not unique to this affliction. Need proof? Just look in the self-improvement section at your local bookstore, or turn on a little daytime television. Flip through the channels any day of the week and two thirds of what you're going to see pouring out at you is how to get more _____. The blank may change from one channel to the other, but the quest, the need to get more, remains universal.

Why do we need more? Well, we need more money so we can get more stuff. For two decades the U.S. economy has been based on a simple principle...consume, consume, consume. When our economy hit a bump and consumer spending dropped the first domino fell, setting off a chain reaction that reverberated around the world.

I hate to admit it, but I'm no different from anybody else. I fall hook, line, and sinker for the lure of the consumer advertisement. I know that they're just shallow manipulations of my individual gullibility. And while I know this intellectually, at some deep basic level, for some reason, I believe what the commercials are telling me.

I need a new Lexus. That three-year-old bomb I'm driving isn't cool anymore. I need the new one. And yes…yes…yes Lord knows I need that new I-pad. I can download three million songs and a thousand movies and…and…and, who knows what else? All I'm sure of is, I'm sure I need one.

Unfortunately, as much as I delude myself into believing it is, my need isn't real. I don't have time to download a hundred movies, much less a thousand. I have three movies on my current tablet, and yet I'm coerced into believing I need a newer, more technically sophisticated model. With the rapidity of technological evolution in the modern world, this cycle of need and fulfillment is never ending. As soon as I buy the new Lexus or I-pad they'll start advertising a newer model. One that fuses both of them and comes with a thought activated cell phone in it. And as soon as I get that, there'll be an even newer model with both the cell phone and a miniature teleportation device, so I can teleport myself, my Lexus, and my I-pad to Tahiti to drive around for only a nominal fee. And so it goes ad infinitum.

In a lot of ways medicine is the same way, but instead of ego and vanity being the primary driving forces, it is our very lives that are at stake. We want more and we want better, the heck with better, we want the best. Who doesn't feel like they deserve the best health care? America is nothing, if not an egalitarian society, in this regard. Everybody deserves the best health care, right?

Well, I don't know. Let me pose a hypothetical scenario. What if there was a drug that was ninety-nine percent effective in preventing osteoporosis in post-menopausal women? And, what if it had no identifiable side effects? Shouldn't we give it to everyone that could benefit from it?

That seems like a "no brainer". And it would be, until you find out that it costs twenty thousand dollars a dose? Ok, well, that does seem a bit steep. But it really would make so many lives better. I guess we still should.

The problem is, at that cost, for that many women, most of which will be sixty-five years old or older, the cost of the drug will bankrupt Medicare in a single year.

Now, should we make this wonder drug available to our Medicare beneficiaries? By the way, I hate the term beneficiaries, almost as much as I hate the term, health care provider. These are patients; sweet little grandmothers and mamas, wonderful women, and you're their doctor and you have this wonder drug that will make their lives so much better. No longer will they have to face the chronic back pain and the debility of nerve root compressions that are associated with the pathologic fractures of osteoporosis. Should you give it to them? And, if you do who should pay for it?

This isn't a medical decision. Medically, the answer is obvious. From a risk-benefit standpoint the drug is amazingly effective, so it's all benefit with no risk. The only risk is to the solvency of the largest health care provider in the United States, Medicare, and by extension the viability of our government as a source for health care coverage for those that have no other way to afford it.

So, this decision becomes not a medical decision but a social decision, a governmental decision, a legal decision, even a moral decision. It is a decision that will reverberate through the years. If the recent financial downturn has shown us anything, it's that consumption has it's limits, and those limits are imposed by the availability of funds. Deficit spending and debt are only sustainable so long as there is someone willing to lend us the money that we don't have. We are currently in a position that requires that we make a decision on how we will impose spending limits because we're running out of credit.

Because our economy is, to say the least, less robust than it was a few years ago and the increasing number of folks becoming Medicare eligible due to the baby-boomers pouring into the over-65 population like water from a busted dam, things can't work like they used to.

We need a better system. Not one dominated by partisan politics, and we need to do it soon. The system we have now is failing and its loss will effect, not just ourselves, but what kind of future we leave for our children.

My Kind of Hunting Story

I'll just let you know right here at the start, that I understand that just from reading the title of this column that a lot of you are going to start off being somewhat skeptical. Now, I'm well aware that most hunting and fishing stories have a tendency to grow in the telling. After a few repetitions they become, to be charitable, exaggerations and some, to be more accurate, turn into outright lies. So, I can certainly understand your skepticism. I want to assure you however, that this isn't that kind of hunting story.

See, the purpose of most of those questionable tales of hunting or fishing prowess is to make the protagonist look good, not just good, but good beyond believability. This story kind of goes the other way, and I can promise you that if I were inclined to exaggerate or lie about this story I would have concocted it in such a way that I came out looking a lot better than I do.

In fact, because this story portrays me in a less than flattering light, I probably wouldn't even be telling it if my good friend Dr. Tony Thomas hadn't asked me to. I prefer to keep my rugged, macho image intact, and avoid any stories that help to make me look like a fool, as I don't generally need all that much help in that particular matter.

Hell, in this story I'm just hoping to come out looking like an innocent victim of circumstances beyond my control. It's kind of sad when that's about the best you can hope for, but even that may be stretching it, as there were several decisions, that in looking back, may not have been quite as good as they seemed to be at the time I made them.

Those of you who know my life circumstances know that Charlene and I have had a kind of revolving door policy on children, although more have tended to come in than have gone out. They come at various times and ages, and we generally don't have much say as to when, but I guess that's okay too. It did get a little strained when four or five showed up in eleven months. Anyway, last year Holton, Charlene's nephew arrived. He was eleven, the same age as our daughter Allison. Now Holton was at a significant disadvantage as far as hunting or shooting were concerned. His dad, who was already deaf, progressively lost his vision to diabetes before Holton was born. His mom developed cancer and died before he was three. So, the sum total of Holton's experience in the outdoors, involved looking out of windows.

Allison on the other hand grew up in a house with four older brothers, who had all, through the years, progressed and moved on into their lives and out of the house. The result though, is that she can drive just about anything with a motor, is the best fisherperson in the house, and can flat-out shoot. With the arrival of youth weekend for deer season, things weren't really going too well, Allison was ready to go, but we couldn't quite get Holton's shooting any where close to the five shots into a paper plate at fifty yards I've always set as a requirement to be able to start deer hunting.

Holton wasn't really all that happy about coming to live here anyway. His father had suffered a stroke and the move was court ordered, to keep him out of a foster home, so the transition was traumatic to say the least. Having a girl cousin that could outshoot him and was going to get to go hunting, while he wasn't, was weighing pretty heavy on an already sad heart.

So, I figured, I made the rules, in this instance I might just have to adjust them. I got a twenty-four by thirty inch box and set it up at the fifty yard line and we started on that. Still, a lot of bullets were hitting dirt on every side of the box, and Allison was pointing out, correctly, and repeatedly, that the problem was flinching, and there was no way he was going to hit a deer jerking the rifle when he pulled the trigger, so we gave up on Allison's .243 and moved down to a .223. With a smaller gun and less recoil, we saw a little improvement, but he was still going to need some work.

We decided to postpone Holton's first hunt a week, to give him some more time. Allison announced that if Holton wasn't going to hunt then she didn't want to hunt either, because they were going to have a contest and the first one of them to get a deer would be the winner, and she wanted to give Holton a chance, so she could beat him fair and square. About this time Maddie, our six year-old daughter piped up, "I want to be in the contest too!"

"Look, baby," I said, "You're too little, besides you don't want to shoot a deer do you?"

"Sure I do," she answered. "Besides I can already shoot better'n Holton, and he's gonna get to go."

Here, I had the great idea that would prove my undoing, "Okay," I said sitting my Styrofoam coffee cup on top of Holton's box, "If you can shoot this cup five times, you can go."

Sitting on my knee in a rocking chair, and leaning the forearm of the rifle on the porch rail, she fired the first shot, knocking the cup off of the box, twice more I reset the cup and she knocked it off the box with the little .223. After the third shot, the cup fell beside the box instead of behind it, and she stopped me when I started to take the gun, "You don't have to walk out there, I can hit it from here." She said. And she did, twice. That made it a three-way contest.

So, that's how I ended up taking three children hunting at the same time. To make matters worse, I decided that we should all hunt in a 4x4 shoot house with a sturdy white plastic chair for me and folding stools for the children. I know you're thinking, "Why would he go and do a ridiculous thing like trying to fit four people, even if three of them were children, in a one man shoot-house?" Well, there was a perfectly good reason. It was the only ground stand we had on the farm. I figured being crowded was a whole lot better than someone (probably me) falling down a ladder from a raised stand.

Just getting us all in there was the first challenge. Those of you who have been deer hunting know that you want to get into the shoot-house and settled with as little noise and distraction as possible, to avoid scaring away any deer that might be near-by. In our case, I would be surprised if we didn't scare away all the deer in Newton County and a good portion of the deer and hogs in Jasper County as well. To say it wasn't very quiet would do it an injustice.

We tried several different variations of how to get all of us in such a small space unsuccessfully. The problem was, that if I put the kids in first, I had to smash them up or step on them to get in myself. Eventually, with a few contortions, we managed to all get in and sit down. I sat down first and the children wedged their stools in around me, adjusting them until somehow we all got in together.

Things were pretty tight for the kids in there and in less than ten minutes the inevitable began.

"Don't touch me!"

"Holton touched me first."

"Maddie's breathing on me."

"Holton's banging his head against the wall, he's gonna scare all of the deer away."

"When will the deer get here? Are they coming now?"

"Why's your face so red daddy? Do deers like it when your face turns red?"

This went on continuously for the next twenty or thirty minutes. At one point, I looked over to see Allison with her head sticking out of the side window of the shoot house.

"What are you doing?" I asked, in my least perturbed voice.

"I can't see good over Maddie. So I thought I could see better, if I stuck my head out the window," she answered.

I guess it made sense to her, so I explained that while she may well be able to see the deer better that way that they would undoubtedly be able to see her better as well. At that point, my systolic blood pressure was at a pretty stable 220. So, to keep from having a stroke, or harming any children, I made the most sensible decision of this whole misadventure.

"Look guys," I started, leaning back in the plastic chair, "Daddy's going to take a nap. Whoever sees a deer first, can wake Daddy up and they can be the one to shoot the deer."

"Like that one standing over there." Maddie piped up.

My eyes followed where her little arm was pointing, and sure enough, there stood an eight-point buck watching us quizzically, tilting his head first one way and then the other, trying to figure what the noisy things in the box were. Immediately, I slid the muzzle of the rifle out of the front window of the shoot house. Here the physics of a two hundred and fifty pound man coming forward onto the cheap plastic legs of a five dollar chair in thirty-five degree temperatures came into play. As the chair came down, the front legs broke off, dumping me face first against the front wall of the shoot house. When that happened, the back legs of the chair sproinged out from under it, and up against the back door, wedging me, neck crooked at seventy-five degrees, between the chair seat and the front wall. So there I was, can't go forward, can't go back, can't move to either side because of the children wedged in around me, can't even move my right arm, for fear of the rifle muzzle coming back into the shoot house with the children.

"Can any of you unlock the door?" I asked, pretending that these kind of things happen when you're deer hunting all the time.

"The latch won't come up, the chairs pushing on the door too hard," Allison answered. "Can you move forward a little?"

Moving forward was not an option, as there was no range of motion left in my cervical vertebrae. When I started getting a little woozy because my carotids were pretty much getting crimped by the angle of my neck, I realized that there was really only one solution. So, that's what I did.

Kicking back, like a mule, as hard as I could, I broke the latch off the door and knocked one of the hinges loose. That let the chair fall backwards out of the house, and off my butt. As I struggled to my knees, I looked out the front window of the shoot house, and across the field, straight at us, came the buck, head bobbing the whole way.

The children could tell something was up by the amazed look on my face, so they too looked out the front window. Holton, unused to the outdoors in the first place, and unaware of my cleverly planned strategy to lure the buck closer, misunderstood the deer's curiosity.

"Shoot him, shoot him, he's chargin'," he screamed, at the top of his lungs.

The buck, taking notice of Holton's flailing arms decided that he had seen enough of this show for one day, and across the fence and into the woods he went.

As we watched the flying white flag that signifies escape, and not surrender Maddie observed. "That sure was a funny deer. Do you think he was deaf, or somethin'?"

"I don't know Mat." I said. "You never can tell.

Maddie and I went back the next night, and the buck returned. She aimed at him, but raised her eyes.

"I don't think I really want to shoot a deer," she said.

"That's okay, do you want me to shoot him?" I asked.

She thought a minute, "Yeah," she answered.

"Are you sure it won't bother you for me to shoot it?" I asked.

"No sir," she said, shrugging her shoulders. "I think he must want to get shot."

Postscript:
    Allison shot her first buck on her own, on our birthday. We share the same birthday and I called home from a hunting trip in Kentucky two days before it to ask her what she wanted for our birthday. Her answer? She wanted us to spend our birthday hunting together. I packed my gear got in my truck and we did. Milliseconds after killing her first buck she killed her second. She shot once and they both fell, dead as stones.

    Holton also got his first buck on his own, this year.

    Maddie is my most frequent hunting partner. After the other two had shot their deer she was relentless. We hunted morning and evening for several weeks in a row. One morning about five forty-five a nice six point walked to the same shoot house we had been in that first day. He came straight in to about ten yards away and just stood there.

    Maddie brought up her gun, but just watched him.

    "Do you want to shoot him?" I whispered.

    "No." She mouthed silently.

    "Do you want me to shoot him?"

    "No." She said. "He's too young and handsome. He needs to grow up and have a good life."

    Maddie and I still hunted after that, but the pressure was off. She'd had the chance. She didn't need to take it. She hasn't killed a deer yet, but we do have a lot of fun watching them through the binoculars. Waiting for that old granddaddy deer that's about to fall over dead of old age.

The Faith of the Moneychangers

I have to tell you that I don't care for prosperity theology. If God wants to give me something, and I'm hoping it isn't an incurable disease, that's between him and me. I don't think nagging him is going to help much. We've all had kids that just wouldn't let something go.

"Can I have it now daddy?...How about now?...Is it time yet?...Can I get it now?"

If you have, you know that while we all still love that child, and we may let them get what it is they've been asking for eventually, there's a reason I'm not sure that's how I want God to feel about me personally.

Lately it seems like I'm in the minority. Between the recent popularity of books like The Prayer of Jabez and preachers of the "gospel of wealth" like Joel Osteen, I'm wondering, if America isn't becoming a nation of moneychangers?

Most Christians are familiar with the story of Jesus driving the moneychangers out of the temple in Jerusalem. Now, when this happened, the Jesus that's portrayed isn't a happy man. He doesn't walk over to the tables and say something like, "Hey you guys are really not suppose to be in here," or "Maybe you and your dove-selling buddies should move your business outside." Nope, what we have here is a very teed-off Jesus. He is affronted by the behavior of these men. Affronted to the point, that this man of divine peace is driven to physical violence. It was notable enough that the description of it is essentially identical in three of the four synoptic gospels.

Can you imagine the scene, benches flying, coins strewn across the ground, doves flopping around and flying up hitting people? And in the middle of it all, Jesus physically chasing these men out the temple door, and then after he had ejected every one of them, he stood, barring the entry to prevent them from returning? No siree, this is not a happy Jesus.

The problem is, I don't think he'd feel much differently today. He made that much effort to show us how he felt, at a time we now refer to as "Passion Week." Knowing that to take this type of action against the "business" of the temple would be the provocation that precipitated his own death, he did it anyway.

It would be harder for him now though. Now the moneychangers aren't in one spot. They're in bookstores, on the Internet, on television, and ministering in huge churches. They give a whole new meaning to the term "false prophet." They won't hesitate to tell you though, that they make no claims to being prophets. They are unconcerned with prophets. It's only the profits that they lay claim to.

The new prosperity theology is based on the same pretexts as its tarnished predecessors. Men like Jim Bakker and Jimmy Swaggart. The new practitioners take the old "send-me your-money" pitch and give it a slight twist and say, "God wants us both to get a bunch of money (or a good parking place, or a good seat at the theater, or any other ridiculous selfish thing they can think of), and we can show you how to get it. All you got to do is..." Anybody smell the snake oil cooking?

Now, I don't mind Christians making a lot of money, or Muslims, or Jews, or Hindus, or anybody else. Buying and selling, owning television or radio stations, good real estate investments are all fine, religious fraud is not.

What bothers me the most intellectually is the idea of taking some minor passages in any book, and using it to alter or pervert the overall message of the entire work. We wouldn't stand for it if the book in question were a medical textbook, or a legal precedent. What makes it okay if it's the bible?

The people doing this aren't too hard to see through if you take the time to go back and read the bible passages they quote. Unfortunately, too few people are doing that, and the people that get hurt worst are the very people who are least capable of that type of discernment and analysis.

Too often today, it's seen as wrong to question any type of religious authority. Especially if what they're saying is accepted as legitimate by the majority. I have to say, that in my humble opinion, that's a load of organic fertilizer. It's never wrong to question wrongdoing.

To me the biggest irony of "prosperity theology" is that the people that are promoting this type of thinking think of themselves as good Christians. They intend, I would suppose, on going to heaven and meeting Jesus. That would be the same Jesus who blocked the temple entrance to keep the moneychangers and dove sellers from turning his father's house into a "den of thieves." Unless he's changed a lot in the last two thousand years, I'm just not sure that they're going to get the reception that they're expecting.

I know a lot of you are wondering why I'm giving you a Sunday-school lesson instead of talking about important stuff. Well, we all have our own moneychangers. In medicine we know its hucksters, frauds, and insurance scammers. In our country it's the "profiteers" who convinced us that it was okay to give mortgages to people that couldn't really afford them. That we should buy beyond our means. That credit card debt doesn't hurt us. That it's okay to lie to investors to prop up stock prices. That it's conceivable that the governments of our world can continue to dole out billions of dollars, or Euros, or pounds to bail every industry that has succumbed to the sirens song of greed.

Right now we have keep our eyes open, our courage intact, and most importantly, we need to remember why it was that Jesus was upset with the moneychangers. It wasn't that they changed one form of currency for another that he minded. It was how much they kept for themselves.

Author's note: There are those who will question my decision to include this piece exactly as it first appeared, as eulogies are not generally included in collections of short stories. I am quite happy that anyone questions this choice, as it means you've read this far, and that in itself is a good thing. I include it, quite simply, because it is the purest, most honest thing I've ever written. sa

Heroes

Between my time as a Navy diver and the years I've spent as a radiation oncologist, it seems like I've spent my entire adult life among heroes, and I'm talking about the real kind, not the kind we see in movies or read about in comic books growing up. The celluloid or comic book kinds don't impress me. As Ray Davies, of the Kinks, sang "...because celluloid heroes never feel any pain, and celluloid heroes never really die." Overcoming pain and facing your own mortality are the very essence of heroism. Who cares if Superman stands in front of a guy with a gun? That's like me being brave enough to swat a mosquito.

I lost one of my heroes last week. He was one of our own, a fellow Mississippi physician, Dr. Mel Flowers. Now Dr. Flowers was a great guy, but I didn't call him Mel. Some people did, but to me it just didn't seem right. When you look at the fifty page CV he left behind with the 42 publications, 67 abstracts, and 112 presentations, you have to be impressed, but they don't tell you much about the man.

For those of you who didn't know him, he was W. Mel. Flowers, Jr., M.D., F.A.C.R. and those last four letters were very important to him, I'll tell you more about that later. He was the head of Nuclear Medicine at University Medical Center and had been part of the University of Mississippi in various forms as an undergraduate, in medical school, as an intern, and as a Radiology resident. He took a little time off to serve in both the Air Force, and Army, but after coming back to start his residency in 1961 he stayed at medical center the rest of his long and distinguished career. These aren't the things that I know about him, they're things I read about.

What I did know about him was that he cared more about teaching Radiology than anybody I've ever met. He understood that education was a never-ending continuum, that you had to keep on teaching and keep on learning, and that the two things were inseparable, teaching begat learning and learning begat teaching. Residents regularly presented at the Mississippi Radiological Society meetings, under Dr. Flowers watchful eye and when they didn't have anything to show us, he did.

He was the keeper of the four letters, F.A.C.R., Fellow of the American College of Radiology. He was the cheerleader for fellowship, telling us regularly that although the requirements were daunting, that being a member of that fellowship signified a singular accomplishment in our field. That only ten percent of radiologists ever attain their goal, usually late in their career, and that to get there we had to get through him. He was the keeper. He only allowed those who were qualified to be nominated, and because he did, those that were nominated were usually picked.

He was a strong supporter of the state medical association encouraging members of the Radiological Society to participate in our state's political and decision making process. It's funny, I can remember how proud I felt, when he walked up to me after one of our meetings, and asked, "So, you're on the Board of Trustees for state?" and when I replied that yes, I was, got a nod and a one word reply. "Good."

I watched through the years as he fought a relentless fight against the malignancy that eventually took his life. I saw the body weaken, the difficulty he had getting into meetings and getting his things arranged, but when he began to talk the voice, weaker, was still resonant and the shine in his eyes as he confounded us with yet another case, was unmistakable. I heard the stories of his being late for work, and when someone checked on him, he was still in his car, too weak to make it into the building without a wheelchair. Yet in the wheelchair he would climb, and be wheeled into his office to teach, and to learn what he could from those he taught.

The last time I saw him, he gave a thirty minute presentation, talked about this year's slate of fellowship nominees, and was genuinely surprised to receive the Mississippi Radiological Society's first Gold Medal for a lifetime of achievement in Radiology.

What can you say when one of your heroes passes away? Well, what I say is...Thanks...Thank you Dr. Flowers...Thanks for everything.

R. Scott Anderson
M.D. F.A.C.R.

Chapter Thirteen

"I don't know if you've been paying attention and I probably shouldn't mention it at all, but this is the thirteenth chapter of this book, so.... Run, run for your life. Skip this chapter and go on over to Confabulation Nation as fast as your page turning fingers can carry you."

"That's a little extreme, don't you think?"

What you should probably do kind of depends on what your phobias are. If you have arachnophobia you're pretty safe, I don't see any spiders around here anywhere. If you have agoraphobia, just stay home and keep reading with the windows shut and you'll be fine. But if you have triskaidekaphobia, well, maybe you'd better go ahead and run on.

Triskaidekaphobia is an unreasonable fear of the number thirteen. It has a history that dates back to ancient times, but the origins of it aren't really all that clear. Some people blame it on the Vikings, well specifically Loki, the troublemaker. He was their thirteenth god. Some people blame it on Judas for being the thirteenth guy to show up at the last supper, and everybody knows how that turned out. Some even blamed it on Hammurabi for leaving out the thirteenth law in his Code way back in 1760 B.C. Although that last one is a load of crap. Some joker named L. W. King, who did the 1910 translation of the Code, just decided that he was entitled to leave off the thirteenth law, the one about debt and inheritance, because he was too superstitious to translate it.

But even with it's convoluted past, one thing is for sure, people are still suffering from it even today. Hotels are missing thirteenth floors, planes are missing thirteenth rows, and some cities are even missing thirteenth streets.

And for the superstitious, if thirteen is unlucky, then Friday the thirteenth is unlucky with a capital U. Well, I'm going to tell you, I'm not one of those. Friday the thirteenth is my lucky day.

"NO...no...no don't lecture me that that's just another reversed superstition. It's not a superstition, it's true. I have iron-clad proof," my right brain huffs.

"What proof?" My left brain asks."

"Our life."

"You know anecdotal evidence doesn't constitute reasonable proof. Now get back to the story and don't stick in a bunch of nonsense."

"Does so, and this _is_ part of the story, it's not nonsense."

"Then get on with it."

Anyway, as I was saying before I was so rudely interrupted. I've thought that Friday the thirteenth was a lucky day, ever since my freshman year in medical school. I'd spent two weeks dreading a Pharmacology exam because we had to take it on Friday the thirteenth. I studied extra hard, but there wasn't any hope I'd do very well on it. I just wasn't getting the material. No matter how much I tried to squeeze it all into my head, every time I looked back over the chapters big bunches of it had leaked out somewhere.

So Friday came as it does every week, and I marched off to face the music like a man headed to the gallows, I was too busy dreading the test to look up and check the crosswalk before I walked into it. The next thing I knew the morning hum was ripped apart by the squeal of rubber on asphalt. I jerked my head up to see a two-ton Pontiac Bonneville coming at me at thirty-five miles an hour. What I found the most puzzling later, when I had time to think about it, was that when I looked up and saw the car bearing down on me the thing that crossed my mind wasn't, "Whoa, I'm about to get squished by a land yacht." It was, "Hey, at least I won't have to take the test." And when the car swerved into the oncoming lane and smashed into a pick-up truck six inches from my left knee, it wasn't relief that I felt, it was anxiety that now I still had to take the damned test. How unlucky could one day be?

It wasn't until I took the test and the material hit all the high spots, just the ones on which my memory shone most brightly, and after that when I knew that I had in fact made a ninety-nine on the examination, that I realized just how lucky I had been not to be killed or maimed on my way to take it.

Confabulation Nation

"I slept wrapped in a veil of dreams. I awoke trapped in a veil of lies."

I've reached the point where I'm never sure what's real on TV anymore. I don't think any of those shows they call "reality shows" are real. It's too obvious that they're scripted. The problem is that half of the time I feel the same way about the news. As a writer, I kind of wish that I had the kind of creativity the guys that write the news have, but I don't. I just can't suspend disbelief the way I used to. It's too obvious that, whoever it is you're watching, that they're only reporting on one side of a thing. I find it incredible that an intelligent audience can accept these things as facts.

It comes down to this very simple question, that's impossible to answer any more. "What is the truth?"

When I first meet my patients I warn them. "I never lie. So be careful about what questions you ask me, because I'll answer them," I say.

But I do lie I guess. Everyone does. I don't think we can help it, because the truth isn't static. It's dynamic, it changes as time passes. The best thing to do for a patient's cancer today probably won't be the best thing to do for the same cancer in five years. We get more facts and KAZAMMM the truth changes.

It doesn't really matter which side you're on, on any subject. Whether you're a democrat or a republican; whether you're a capitalist or a communist; whether you're an Arab or a Jew, there's never been a shortage of wild ideas about the truth. And the truth for one group may be impossible to believe for the other.

As far as I understand, the truth is supposed to be the facts of whatever it is that happened. Not the way what happened gets manipulated to sound a certain way. Spin, is what they call manipulating the truth on television. You can spin a fact so that it can support whatever it is you want, or attack whatever it is you don't want. In the age of television, spin is the name of the game. The same facts presented on Fox News, CNN, or on MSNBC, somehow, turn out to be completely different truths.

So, how can we, just plain old people, see through all of this whirly manipulation of the facts? First, we have to admit that it's being done, and then we have to see that it happens on both sides of every argument.

We can always spot the spin if we disagree with it. It's always easy to come up with a laundry list of ridiculous statements presented as fact, when someone you don't like makes them. Now, in general, when this happens we don't have any trouble with how we feel about it. We just go ahead and call it a lie, and once we call it a lie we don't have a whole lot of interest in being contradicted.

We don't look quite as hard at misrepresentations of stuff we're supporting as long as that misrepresentation remains positive. But wait and see how mad we get at the news media for pointing out anything negative about whatever it is we support.

Why are we like this? Why are they like this? If it's the other side, it's because they're no-good rotten liars. If it's our side it's because of the no-good rotten media, or a right wing conspiracy, or whatever we can think of to shake our fist at.

The problem is that we start to believe in stuff. We start to think that this thing or that thing is right, and we start getting involved in bending the truth. We don't even usually do it on purpose. Mostly it's just because we forget to label the stuff that's really just an opinion as opinion. That's because we start to believe that there are "right" opinions. Then it gets hard to tell what's fact and what's opinion.

Any statement that relies too heavily on emotion is usually an opinion. If you're saying something is good, or something is bad, you have to watch out. Almost nothing is all good or all bad either.

As my mother used to say, "There're two sides to every story."

"It was not the monarchy or the needs of the people of France that

was the pain in the delicate little neck of Marie Antoinette. Both sides had valid points. The argument was decided not by the points of debate but by the pointed edge of the guillotine's blade."

Whichever side you believe, poor Marie lost her head, not just because of her political opinions, but because the folks on the other side of the argument believed in theirs enough to kill her. They were sure she was bad. They knew it emotionally. They believed it viscerally. They acted on that belief lethally. The same kind of thing happened to a guy named Jesus.

So, why is it that we're all so all-fired sure we know the answers all of the time? It isn't because we're bad people, and it isn't because the other guys are bad people either (although sometimes they are). It's just that the two sides exist in alternative intellectual realities. They take the same set of facts and believe in different truths.

If you subscribe to the notion that the future offers infinite possibilities, and that the past is solid and immutable, then the present is like a zipper, fusing all of those possibilities as it passes. We can't really know the truth about the future, until we get there. The present is too immediate. We can only know what is happening to our self as an individual. So, your only source of clues is the past, and there's the problem. You have to know what the past truly was. An old saw says that history is written by the winners, and to a large extent that's true. But an equally big problem is that we can't know what we can't see. We're stuck with the opinions and prejudices of the persons who recorded whatever it is we're looking at. To know the truth, we have to look for the falsehoods.

"*I have wondered for the longest time whether everybody knows they're lying, or it's just that nobody knows what in the world the truth is.*"

There are three kinds of untruth: lies, which are deliberate untruths; fantasies, which are more like wishes, but are easily distinguished by the fact that the person doing the fantasizing knows what the truth is;

and then there's confabulation. For those of you that don't have a DSM 238, or whatever edition they're up to now (alright, I know you think I'm confabulating on the number, but this is just an example of literary license, because I'm too lazy to look it up), confabulation is a condition in which a patient, usually due to an organic condition, like Munchausen's syndrome, Korsakoff's syndrome, or any number of organic maladies, doesn't know what the truth of their past is, because they're unable to remember it.

To compensate for their lack of memory, they simply make something up. Munchausen's syndrome describes elaborate and fantastical untruths that are made up to fill in the void in the patient's memory. I'll give you an example. You see that one of the patient's knees is scraped, so you ask, "What happened?" They respond with a story in which an asteroid hit the earth's surface, cracking the earth's crust, and releasing a fiery plume that shot three hundred feet into the air. At the apex of the plume a dragon formed, and flew down to terrorize the city. "Amazing," you reply. "But that doesn't explain what happened to your knee." They give you a confused look, and then say, "Well I guess I skinned it when I ran away."

You see, I believe that's what explains a lot of all those crazy opinions we hear on TV. Some folks may very well be liars, and I'm sure some of them are fantasizing. But for the most part, I think they're just making it up, because they don't know what the truth is. Most of us aren't ardent students of history, and most of us will never know the facts we want to about the past, because our historical records have holes in them. The same kind of holes the patient with Munchausen's syndrome has in his memory, and that's why we have no choice <u>but</u> to confabulate.

Judaism is such a durable religion, because it took advantage of a peculiarity of the human brain. People can remember words set to music verbatim much more easily than they can remember words told as stories. The Cantor gave them the edge until writing came along. They were also the first religion to codify its beliefs in written form. Hinduism, Buddhism, Christianity and Islam followed suit. Each of these religions has a common set of beliefs that they hold to be true, they differ from one another because some of the facts that they hold true differ. Who's wrong? Who's right? Who knows?

We'd all probably get along a lot better if we recognized our mutual confabulation. That James Frey guy wouldn't have gotten hollered at by Oprah if he'd have just started out saying, when he wrote his memoir/novel/fantasy/confabulation/lie, "When I wasn't high or drunk, for the most part, I didn't have a pencil handy. So this is about the best I can remember."

You can, however, get into trouble if you dismiss the things your patients tell you as confabulation, unless they're talking about dragons, and even then you may want to consider detox first. Your patients, for the most part, are giving you important facts, even when they're giving you an opinion. "The pain is really bad," isn't offering a value judgment on pain itself, but is an attempt to quantify the amount of pain that they actually have. Even if they tell you, "I'm having this pain in my head, it started last week, but you know, my aunt told me that my momma dropped me on my head when I was a baby, and I think that's what's probably to blame," you better listen. They have a new onset of headache. Causality may suffer, but the incident facts are usually true.

"If facts and numbers are the food with which we nourish our minds, quotations and statistics are simply the garnish by which we change the look of the plate."

The past may be immutable, but it is also, in many ways, unknowable. None of us really know the truth of our existence any more than the proto-hominoids of mankind's distant past a million years ago or so ago did. None of us knows the future.

Five million years from now the sun may evolve and its form, due to the consumption of hydrogen and the increase in its gravity, will cause it to heat up and burn off the earth's atmosphere, when that happens, all of earth's water may dry up and then the earth's crust may melt, we could turn to a giant ball of molten lava. Now, that's global warming worse than Al Gore ever thought about.

Why would I think such a thing? Well, there are people who

support that scenario based on astrophysical observation and statistical extrapolation. And it could be true, but it's just as likely that it's simply some scientist, sitting in a laboratory, confabulating away. I'm guessing that I won't be there to find out anyway, and I don't guess my children will be either.

What I'm trying to say, is that we should all try and be a little more understanding with each other, because we're all suffering from the same disease, mortality. None of us has been here long enough to know the truth of hardly anything, so we should be more gentle with each other, because, we're all doing the best we can, just making it up as we go along.

All of the quotes used in this article are really quite nice little quotations that I just made up to illustrate the point that quotations are the very kinds of opinions that are wielded as facts to support an argument. Even if I wrote:

"$E=mc^2$" _{A. Einstein}

that is the case. Yes subsequent measurements and experiments have supported the equation, but when Einstein wrote those five figures they were quite simply Albert's opinion.

According to Plan

Most of you have heard me talk about my wife. Well, not literally, but, you've read about her here in this space for the last little while, and if you did you probably remember that we have a kind of an unusual family. I know a lot of you think the same thing about your own family, and those of you who don't, may be wearing blinders on that particular subject. Our family is unusual in that it grew with some twists and turns we never expected.

When I graduated from medical school, we were supposed to put our favorite quote on the yearbook page with our senior picture. There were quotes from doctors, quotes from Freud, quotes from Nietzsche, all kinds of stuff. The quote I chose was a lyric from a song by John Lennon. "Life is what happens to you while you're busy making other plans." Boy-oh-boy, when I chose that I never guessed how true it was going to turn out to be, especially when it came to Charlene.

Char and I spent the first year of our marriage on Coronado Island on a narrow strip of land about one-hundred yards wide, called the Coronado Cays, with San Diego harbor outside our front door and the Pacific Ocean outside our back. Our biggest decision was where we were going to sit and drink our glass of wine after dinner, listening to the clink and clank of the rigging of the sailboats, or the rhythmic crashing of the waves. We didn't have any money, but we didn't care much. We were living in a house we could never afford, in a neighborhood with Orville Redenbacher and Michael Jordan as neighbors. Charlene got us the house. A breast cancer patient we were treating was a realtor, with a unique specialty; she took care of wealthy people's homes. She had come up with a great solution to rot and vandalism. She had young married naval officers, without children, live in the houses as caretakers. So, we got a part-time job living in President Regan's ambassador to South Africa's house.

It was wonderful, until the U.S.'s relationship with South Africa, was terminated over the apartheid issue. Then one day the ambassador, his wife and crew sailed up to the slip outside the front door, on a fifty-four foot open-water cruiser, and offered us a bunch of money to vacate the premises post-haste. I guess that was the end of the honeymoon. It was just as well, while we were waiting to get out, two of the biggest earthquakes to hit San Diego in a century hit four hours apart. When our neighbor explained to Charlene that there wasn't really any use in worrying about the earthquakes, because, if the Strand fault breached, the Cays would be six-hundred feet under water in about six seconds, that was the end of our relaxing days on Coronado.

A year later we were in Meridian, Mississippi. Neither of us is from Mississippi. The ambassador's wife knew a young senator from Mississippi named Trent Lott, who happened to be visiting California. He also happened to be the head of the senate appropriations committee. When Senator Lott asked the Secretary of the Navy if Mississippi could borrow one of the Navy's radiation oncologists, because Mississippi needed one, I was on my way east. Do you see how life keeps happening, just the way I didn't plan?

The thing that kept nagging at me when we first moved here was, why were we looking at four-bedroom houses to buy? We didn't have any children. I should have taken that as a sign. That's when the urge to nest, reproduce, and nurture swept my poor wife over a cliff. A baby (she only admitted to wanting one) became the holy grail of our existence. Now at first, I will admit, I was a more than willing participant, but as endometriosis, became infertility, recreational activities gave way to IVF, GIFT, and I'm not sure how many other initials. It was during this period that Dylan, my son came to live with us. He was seven. He wasn't her baby, heck, he wasn't even a baby at all, but you couldn't tell her that. The un-athletic city girl immediately became a sports mom. She would try whatever sport the season fit, in the yard every day after school. She broke fingers throwing footballs, twisted ankles playing basketball, and landed on her butt more than once tripping on a soccer ball. Still she prayed for a baby.

The IVF's worked, but the pregnancies failed. The GIFT procedures produced embryos, but they wouldn't implant. Eventually, we decided to adopt a child, and even the first few of those fell through. Still she prayed.

Then the dam broke.

We adopted a newborn, Allison at the same time that Charlene's sister Synova had her third little boy Holton, and the two sisters were ecstatic, until Synova was diagnosed with colon cancer. As the cancer progressed despite treatment, Synova's husband, who was already deaf, became totally blind. Life was not happening according to plan.

My oldest son Jackson came to live with us, he was fifteen. Synova died, and her husband suffered a stroke shortly afterward, and Charlene got pregnant with Maddie. In an eleven-month span we got five children. I told Charlene to stop praying for any more.

The moral of this story is that you just never know what life's going to give you. You've got to roll with the punches. Sometimes you need a little help. Every kid came with their own suitcase full of problems. Well, maybe not Maddie. Her biggest problem was that with all of those big brothers, her feet didn't get to touch the ground until she was three-years-old.

Charlene's answer was counseling, with our big mixed bag family, somebody was always fighting with somebody else. So, we went to counseling in every possible combination. It must have worked. No one was killed by a sibling or an angry father. It may have been close some times, but they've all survived so far.

Counseling was a revelation for me. I found out that virtually everything that happened to anybody was my fault. That goes with being a dad. It's a tough job. I can remember how furious the boys would get when I came up with some great mutual punishment that forced them to work together. I always told them the same thing. The world's a tough place and you'd better learn to work with people, if you like them or not, because you're going to have to work with some people you don't like sometime.

With four boys from twelve to seventeen I gained the reputation at the local school as the meanest dad in the universe. I hope it stays that way. I've got two girls coming along.

I've heard that the number one cause of premature deaths in physicians is suicide. In my mind, any death, which involves me personally, I consider premature. I can tell you one thing, if I do turn up dead call in the medical examiner to look for bullet holes, because somebody killed me. I'm not going anywhere if I can help it. See, life's like watching one of those cliffhanger movies. I can't go anywhere. I don't know how it's going to turn out.

Where I Fit in the Food Chain

This year I will have been a parent for thirty years. By itself that doesn't sound like such a big deal. After all, here in the United States, where childhood mortality is relatively low, being a parent for thirty years is, for the most part, simply a matter of the passage of time. Well, you also have to be able to restrain the urge to kill them as teen-agers for all of the stupid stuff they get into. Which, when you think back on all the stupid stuff they got into, is in itself, a minor accomplishment. But that's not what I'm getting at. My point is, that with seven kids spread across twenty years I've been in a state of suspended parenthood for almost all of my adult life. With that being the case, it should come as no big surprise that over that period of time I've seen just about every Disney cartoon ever made. And I'll tell you the truth. I like almost all of them.

But I can't blame my children for my introduction to the Magic Kingdom. I am, like a lot of us baby-boomers, a member of the first Disney generation. I grew up watching *Spin and Marty*, and sang along with Cubby and Annette when the Mickey Mouse Club was the best thing on TV.

The kingdom of the Mouse has, since my childhood, expanded from Los Angeles to Orlando, and today sucks in more money than we have to spend in our entire state every day of the year. Since 1955 we have watched Disney evolve from Mickey Mouse and Donald Duck to Hannah Montana and the Jonas Brothers. The High School Musical series has made more money in a shorter time than anything Disney has ever done in the past. They can generate all that money simply because my generation and the kids that came along after us were willing to accept the idea that a bunch of cartoon animals, or animals in general, could be capable of human reason and interaction. Ascribing human thoughts and emotions to animals is called "anthropomorphism" and it's become so common in our culture that none of us even notice that we're doing it anymore.

But there are side effects to having a whole generation of Americans growing up watching a talking mouse every Sunday night. We've, as a culture, developed a completely unrealistic view of animals in the process.

No more of the old "Kipling era" view of nature as "red in tooth and claw." Sure old Rudyard wasn't above a little anthropomorphisising himself, and the Disney folks seized on it, and gave us their own take on *The Jungle Book.* The end result of all of these years of overexposure to such a huge array of sweet and beguiling animal stories is that, here in America, we've developed a belief in the existence of a bunch of benevolent wildlife that can't wait for us to come and interact with them.

Now, we know that we have to watch out for the occasional bad actor, there are always villains, aren't there? There has to be a bad guy. But we've learned, from years of exposure, to recognize them as soon as they appear on the screen.

In fact, here are a couple of tips for recognizing animal types that are usually bad. Sharks are a prime example. We know that, as a species, sharks simply aren't trustworthy. If you need independent verification of this you have to do no more than watch *Finding Nemo*. Sharks may act friendly at first, but… Besides they aren't even mammals. You just can't really trust any of those "lower species" anyway, not spiders, not snakes, well none of them really.

But, if we're talking about mammals that's a bit harder. While most mammals are friendly and heroic there can be the occasional villain there as well. Just think of Simba and Scar.

Everybody who has kids has seen *The Lion King,* probably a lot more times than they care to. I think at one point between it playing in the car, the playroom, the den, and the kitchen, Allison Hines played the thing four or five times a day. We even had to go to New York and see it on Broadway. Over time, this becomes a "hakuna matada" brainwashing technique.

So, what's the harm in persisting in our little cultural fantasy? None really, as long as we stay in an urban environment and away from the actual animals we think of so fondly. You stop seeing lions as three-hundred pound carnivores with two-inch long teeth and three-inch claws, designed to help provide the twenty-five pounds of red meat a day a grown lion requires to be properly nourished, and start seeing them as singing, frolicking characters that would gladly switch over from killing other mammals and fill up on a bunch of bugs and worms if someone, maybe a meerkat and a warthog, only showed them how to do it. This isn't a particular danger if you stay on Broadway, or in Anaheim, or in Orlando, but it can become a real problem really quickly if you're somewhere, say, like Africa.

It was during the height of *Lion King* mania that I went to Africa for the first time. What all this brainwashing does that's most dangerous, is that it has a tendency to blunt your natural fear of predators. Humans, since the first human watched as his pal Oook was eaten by a saber-tooth tiger, have had a healthy fear of large carnivores. It was a learned behavior from practical experience. It is an experience that most of us in the south have never been exposed to. Growing up in the south, about the only thing we were afraid of in the woods was snakes, because we didn't have any predators left that may have once looked on humans as a potential dinner.

At the beginning of my trip all of my unrealistic expectations were made worse by meeting Maggie, the cheetah that had been raised from a cub, and Ruthie, the warthog that one of the dogs had brought home still alive when she was just a piglet. These were the first animals I came into contact with when I arrived in Africa, they were wild appearing animals, but were, in fact, friendly gentle house pets, and they made you ready for a great time with the friendly African wildlife.

One thing I can tell you for sure, Africa is not a land to be walking around in, in an anthropomorphic stupor. During those first days riding around the countryside we all noticed that most of the houses outside of the cities had seven-foot chain link fences around them. There were three of us from Mississippi there together, and none of us could figure it out.

When we asked the PH (professional hunter) why, he looked at us as if we were idiots before answering, "So, the children don't get eaten, of course."

Now if you're from Meridian Mississippi the idea of a yard fence stops at about five feet. Why you would possible need a seven-foot fence around your yard to keep your kids safe is kind of hard to get your head around. "But, why do they have to be so tall?" I asked.

"Two reasons," he said, and then paused for a few beats to enhance the drama. "Leopards and lions."

Even at my anthropomorphic worst, this sunk in to the bone. These children didn't have the luxury of seeing old Simba as a pal. If he was hanging around, it wasn't because he wanted to sing a few verses of *Hakuna Matada* with the kids, nope, he was there for some chow. I suddenly realized that Simba wouldn't have the slightest reservation about eating me either. To a lion, I wouldn't be much different than one of the kids behind the fences, a high-protein snack, devoid of hoofs, horns, scales, or any other form of natural protection.

"Oh come on, cut the drama," I can hear you say. "The PH was only giving you the old tourist treatment."

And, I might have thought the same thing, but it was the eyes of the children behind the fences that made me a believer. They watched with an intensity you don't often see here, and the eyes of the older ones with the babies on their hips and their eyes scanning the bush any time they left their enclosures. They knew what I was just learning…their place in the food chain. Humans may be at the top of the food chain in most parts of the world, but in Africa, that isn't always the case. Any doubts I may have had left about that would be wiped away completely over the coming days.

My first lesson came after a morning spent in thick thorn-bush. We had walked steadily for about three hours after leaving the truck, and had seen only glimpses of animals in the dense vegetation. We became aware of the sound of something moving, almost dragging itself through the brush, so we got behind an ant hill on the small game trail we were traveling along. In a few minutes a huge hartebeest bull came into view, but something was wrong with the way that it was moving, it would jerk and when it did the brush behind it would bend and sway. It was moving slowly and blood was streaming down its shoulders on both sides. Through the binoculars we could see that it had been caught in a poachers snare. Apparently it had been strong enough to manage to escape by breaking the wire of the snare but in doing so the cruel wire had cut the poor animals neck to the bone. The wire had broken so that he still drug a long length of the wire behind him, and it was now tangled with branches and grass, causing it to cut further into his flesh with every step.

This was a shot that every hunter understands. It was a shot that had to be made, for the sake of the animal. So we had to keep on its trail, going deeper and deeper into the bush, but the animal was hurt and cautious, so it was nearly impossible to get a clear shot. Finally I climbed onto a broken anthill, steadied the rifle on the professional hunter's shoulder and downed the injured buck as it came into a small clearing.

Now, we had done what needed to be done, but we were about half of forever away from the truck. There were two choices, carry the four hundred and fifty pound animal along the twisting game trails or go and try to find a way back here with the truck. The answer was obvious to the guides as they would be the ones that would be carrying the bull. So, while the rest of the party went back to get the truck and all of the tools we needed to load the carcass, I stayed with the hartebeest, to keep the scavengers away. The PH left with the guides, because they were going to need every pair of eyes possible to watch the trail markers that they would leave on the way back. Before he left, he checked that I still had some water left in my canteen, and left me with a final set of instructions.

"It may take a little while, so sit back and relax, but don't go to sleep. Keep an ear out for the truck, and when you hear it, tie your shirt to your gun barrel, then climb up as high as you can on the ant hill, and wave like crazy, so we can find you."

Now, you may not believe this, but in a situation like this, I'm not really that brave of a person. Every time I've ever done anything remotely dangerous, I'm scared. The only times I've ever done anything that anyone else considered brave, I can assure you that it was a complete accident.

Sitting there as the afternoon passed and the sun got nearer and nearer to the horizon my mind wandered, I guess because it was bored, trying to make me crazy by imagining any number of unpleasant outcomes to this little adventure. In the daylight I was sitting next to what anyone would consider excellent bait and a fresh blood trail leading straight to where I was sitting. I had less than five feet of visibility thanks to the dense brush and I could only assume that the visibility would get a lot worse when darkness fell.

The chances of finding my way out of where I was before dark were infinitesimal. I was in the middle of an area I hadn't been in before and I had no idea of where I was, or how to get back to the road. My only option was to wait it out.

For some reason I began to have a bit of anxiety. I am not proud to tell you that I was on top of that anthill for quite a while before I heard the jeep. In Africa I was just meat, just another link in the food chain.

I came back to camp more than a little disappointed with myself. I was no great white hunter. I was, in fact, much closer to Francis Macomber than Robert Wilson.

My second lesson came two days later. The fence around the compound had an area in a low spot where it formed a right angle to follow the contour of the land. It was a great place to use as a trap. Apparently, one of the local lions that had figured that out.

Every day as we drove in and out of the compound we saw a large group of eland antelope. Eland are huge animals, and a fully-grown cow weighs close to two thousand pounds. One of those was easy to recognize as being a constant from day to day Her horns rose and crossed, earning her the nickname of Mrs. X. She was the largest cow in the group and this year had given birth to twin calves.

As we left camp that morning we saw her standing alone on the small hill above the bend in the fence. Our driver turned and we drove in her direction to see if we could see the calves. As we approached we saw jackals ghost up and away from the approaching truck. That was not a good sign. At the top of the rise warthogs ran grunting away from a crimson profusion of blood and in the center was what was left of the two calves. It was hard to tell how much had been eaten by the lion and how much had gone to feed the scavengers, but most of the meat had already been stripped away. Somehow, the lion had managed to trap both of the calves in the corner and kill them both before they could escape. It was almost unbelievable.

It was apparently unbelievable to Mrs. X as well. For the next two days she stood on that hill waiting for one of her calves or the other to come back. Then one afternoon we returned with a good gemsbok and she wasn't there. As we pulled to the skinning shed to unload the buck, there she was hanging on the rack, her crossed horns dragging the ground.

She'd been killed by the lion in the same place, in the same corner, in the same way. The difference was that everyone in the compound had heard this attack, and rushed to respond. They never saw the lion. They'd only heard it.

By the time the trucks arrived Mrs. X was all that remained, her neck ripped open and blood all around. Her size hitting the fence at a full run, followed by her death throes as the lion attacked had resulted in a four foot split in the chain-link.

The idea of a lion killing something of that size was incredible in itself and the fact that it had devised a way to use the fence, as a "tool", was fantastic. I felt a need to keep something of that. Something so unusual demanded proof. So without thinking about it, I left my rifle in the truck and grabbed my camera to go down and take pictures.

Keeping your eye up to a camera eyepiece without keeping an eye on what's around you is never a good idea. I would probably have been chewed up fairly vigorously, if not for pure dumb luck.

While I held the camera through the fence to take pictures, I noticed a juvenile male lion stalking me, so I moved the camera to get a shot of him. It was some bizarre form of disassociation, I knew that he was clearly stalking me, but I was somehow detached, I saw him but I couldn't think of what I should do, so I snapped the shot. Immediately, I noticed a flash out of the corner of my eye and automatically fell back away from the fence, just as a second lion, one that I had never seen, hit the fence, right where I had been standing. Laying there on my back I drew my only weapon, a hunting knife with a five-and-three-quarters inch blade, hoping neither lion had figured out that they could easily push through the break in the fence and get to my side.

I looked at the knife and then back at the lion, as it chewed on the chain-link with what appeared to be a whole mouth full of weapons a lot more dangerous than my little steel claw. The leg of my pants was soaked with the blood of the gemsbok I'd shot that morning. I was hoping that mine wouldn't be mixing with it in the next couple of seconds.

Laying on the ground I was prey. So I stood. I stood and raising my voice shouted as loud as I could. I shouted at them, I shouted for help. I shouted that there were two lions trying to get through the fence.

Luckily that was enough. The lions were afraid of the activity in the compound as people rushed down the hill to see what was going on. They both took off without pushing the issue. I never saw the original lion leave. He just kind of wasn't there the next time I looked for him. I will admit that my attention had been somewhat dominated by the closer lion as he was only about eighteen inches from my feet.

After that, I knew that bravery wasn't an issue when it came to lions. There was no chance I would have survived an encounter with these two lions out in the thick thorn brush with the hartebeest. I know to this day, that even with the .416 rifle in my hands, sitting on the anthill, ready to shoot the lion that I could see stalking me, that the second lion would have gotten me before I could ever have made the shot, and somehow, that was right. That's what hunting should be. It's what a fair chance means. You're never sure who dinner will be. Paraphrasing an old saw "sometimes you eat the lion an' sometimes the lion eats you."

I'm not so sure I'd be all that happy to have to eat a lion, but I will say, I'm really glad it didn't go the other way either. Hakuna matada my butt.

Creative Writing

I got thrown for a loop the other day. One of the girls in the Tumor Registry sent a copy of the JOURNAL version of *Squirrel Story* to the inspector from the American College of Surgeons that was coming to do our cancer center certification. She had great intentions. She wanted to show him how well rounded we were. I understand that and I'm happy for it. That's not what threw me. What did that was what the inspector said the morning he showed up.

He was from Pennsylvania, and I guess up there they don't put goofballs writing about squirrels in their medical journals. But what he said was, that it was amazing that they would included something like *Squirrel Story* in a scientific journal at all, but that he could understand it because this was Mississippi, and Mississippi had such a rich literary tradition that it made sense for it to be there.

That was just the thing to send me into a full-fledged neurotic meltdown.

At my age, I've spent most of my life trying to figure out what good writing is supposed to be. I've spent a lot of time studying it. Reading authors that are recognized as being good writers. I'm starting to get a fair idea of what people say really great writing is supposed to look like, and, how great writers are suppose to write. Unfortunately, I've also come to the unavoidable conclusion that I'm not one of them.

Lord knows, I've tried to be a better writer, but, all of that thrashing around trying to say things in as convoluted and descriptive a manner as possible is exhausting. Not only that, but when I do take the time to go to all that trouble what I end up with is something I don't even like to read.

I know, I know, you're supposed to grow and develop as you keep on, but every time I try to grow, what I write doesn't sound like me anymore. It sounds like me trying to be an idiot is all. The other problem is it's as boring as hell.

I tried reading some Hemingway again, to give me an idea of where I should go. Everybody knows that he's a great writer, and it's been years since I've tried to read any of his short stories. Not because I have anything against him, <u>but he is dead</u>, and he hasn't been coming out with very many new books lately, at least not since his demise anyway. If I remember right from college, the book on Earnest was that what made him revolutionary was a return to the use of short direct sentence structure. Problem is, where the sentences are going is anything but.

Why can't we just have people with names in the stories who were just doing something, without their past crowding them around to the point that you can't tell what they were doing in the first place? Over time it's gotten worse.

Lord knows, I'm not picking on anyone, but since then, modern short story writers can't seem to tell a story. They get so tied up with descriptions and feelings that they forget to tell the story. It's kind of like a flash of lightning at night. And while that sort of thing can be intriguing, to me it's never quite enough. I like to have some idea of what it is I'm seeing. Maybe I lack imagination. But the flavor of the story comes from a little bit of chewing, not simply the quick swallow. Some of it comes from knowing where the proper starting point is, and going on until you reach the stopping point. Every author is going to come up with a different starting point and a different stopping point, but that's okay, as long as you get enough in it to make the reader say, "I like that," and not "What the hell was that?"

There is a natural pressure here to want to try and become a better writer. It's the expectation of the place. Like the inspector from Pennsylvania said, Mississippi has a rich storytelling tradition. You can say anything you want about the relative merits and literary skills of our writers, but by gosh, they've always known how to tell a story.

Something about that makes it hard to be a writer who just so happens to be in Mississippi. There's a lot to live up to. Even saying the name Faulkner is enough to make anything I write seem worthless by comparison. When you throw in names like Eudora Welty, Willie Morris, Ellen Gilchrist, and modern writers like Grisham and Iles that can turn into an absolute creative paralysis. These are all writers that can tell a powerful story, a story powerful enough to be worth remembering for generations.

It was scary enough for me that I wrote both of my first two novels based in someplace other than Mississippi. Just to keep from having to face it.

I think from now on, especially in this little column, I'm just going to have to give up on trying to be some kind of a "Mississippi writer" and just keep on telling my little stories. Who knows? Some of them may even end up being worth remembering, for now anyway.

Teary Sockets

The Story of County 60

    Some of you may have heard that I made a movie last year. I did, and it almost killed me, so did my wife.

    I don't really know how we came up with the whole idea of a movie set almost entirely on a dilapidated old school bus, that's shot half in Los Angeles and half in Mississippi, but we did. I guess we thought that since we didn't have very much money for sets and location fees, that we could save a lot of money if we just shot everything on the bus. Luckily, I have a couple of really good friends that I thought could help us. They're brothers, David and M.L. Waters, but more importantly to where this story is going, they happen to own Waters International and sell school buses. I figured that would be the place to start.

    With just a little bit of looking they were able to find exactly what I'd asked them for. A used short bus, with wheelchair access doors, but with all of the seats removed and the wheelchair access lift removed. These things were important because we were going to be shooting a movie inside the thing. We needed as much access as possible from the outside, and complete freedom in how we configured the interior. The high ceiling gave us room up above to keep the boom mikes out of our shots, and the steps up from the standard school bus doors gave us a place for the Director of Photography to stand with the camera locked down to the handrail, to shoot.

    It was perfect, and it was just the right price, cheap. Now we just had to get a similar bus out in California. There's where the first problem came in. Short buses are pretty unique, at least old ones are. There are so many variations of chassis, coachwork, and door configuration that we were never going to get another one to match. So we made the decision that we were just going to have to get by with only one bus. We'd just take it to

California with us.

The first thing we had to do was, go get the bus. County 60 was four hundred miles away in Tennessee. The first thing my friend David told me was to have the seller deliver the bus to his lot. That way, if something went wrong in transit it would be their problem to deal with, not mine. That certainly seemed to be the smartest thing to do, but we were in kind of a hurry, and the seller wouldn't be able to deliver her for a week. We really needed to get her to Meridian as soon as possible to start her transformation from empty hulk to rolling movie studio. So my two oldest sons Jackson and Dylan left in my GMC 2500 to make the trip. They'd ride up together and then Dylan, in my truck would follow Jackson, driving the bus, home. At least that was the plan. And everything went according to plan 97.625% of the way.

Just nineteen miles from home, four hundred yards across the state line in Alabama, the bus came to a steaming halt.

"Did you check the coolant before you left?" Was the first thing I asked when the boys called.

"Of course we did, but it wouldn't have mattered anyway." Jackson answered, knowing County 60 was going to need some serious work, and not a bottle of antifreeze. "Coolant and oil are running out of the bottom of the engine, all over the ground."

"I'll send a wrecker, and be there in a few minutes." I said.

Going east on the interstate a mile inside Mississippi I passed the boys in my truck, followed by County 60 on the wrecker going west. I made a U-turn in the median just across the state line and saw the huge puddle of antifreeze and oil where the bus had been.

"At best it's got to be a blown head gasket…please let it just be a blown head gasket." I pleaded.

When I got back to town and met the wrecker, I found that my prayers had not been answered. The folks at Waters had already made arrangements with another shop to replace the cracked engine block. So much for the idea that we might get by with just a gasket. Suddenly the extra week it would have taken the seller to deliver the bus didn't really seem that long at all.

We ended up losing a week anyway. The new engine cost more than the bus did to start with. But, at least the thing had a new engine. There couldn't be any reason in the world why we couldn't just drive to California now, could there?

Two days later with Jackson behind the wheel County 60 was heading west. She made it all the way to Newton, Mississippi, thirty-five miles west to be precise, before she started to cut out and had to be brought back. This time it was the alternator that was the culprit. The good news was that, that only took two days before Jackson and the yellow bus were again heading west. They made it to Newton again. This time it was the transmission losing transmission fluid.

Four times the bus left for California, and not once did it make it past Newton. After spending three times the initial cost of the bus, and never even making it forty miles west, I came to the conclusion that there was absolutely no chance that the thing would ever make it to Los Angeles under its own power.

There was only one answer; we were going to have to tow it. We were running out of time. We had an entire film crew that would be waiting to start filming in one week, and they were going to have to be paid if the bus made it or not. So we divided up our resources. The assistant director and the Director of Photography would have to start filming without us, and Jackson, the director, and I, the producer would haul the damned bus across the country.

Now finding something you can haul a school bus on seems a whole lot easier than it actually is. They're too wide for anything designed to haul cars, too heavy for front wheel type trailers, and have too much overhang to pull up on a flatbed. Of course, I didn't know any of these things. We had to learn them all the old-fashioned way, also known as the hard way…trial and error. Ours was a little more error than trial.

I threw caution, and money to the wind, and bought a twenty-six foot goose-neck flatbed trailer, hooked it to my GMC, parked it on a hill, and with a whole lot of scraping, and the loss of about a quarter inch of rear bumper on the part of the bus, forced the bus up the ramp onto the trailer.

Since the overall theme of this exercise seemed to be, "Learning Your Limitations," we went straight back to Waters to get some quick tips on how in the hell we were supposed to keep the bus on top of the trailer. Everybody there was wonderful. We had chains, we had nylon webbing, we had fire extinguishers, and jacks, and mirror extensions and everything we never had any idea that we needed, before we left there. They gave us tips for backing, tips for fueling, tips on just about everything I could think of and a bunch of stuff I hadn't. But the best advice we got before we left I didn't listen to.

"You know you don't have to do this," my friend David said seriously. "There are people who are professionals at doing this. You should leave this to them. You're going to end up saving time and money in the long run, if you let somebody else do it."

This was the second time I didn't listen and the second time he was right on target.

So we left Meridian with the front of the bus chained down with a logging chain and binder, and as much else secured in place with nylon tie-down straps as we could. Now apparently the bus didn't like being tied down, because it broke four or five tie–down straps before we made it to Dallas. The bed of the pick-up looked like a snake pit there were so many pieces of the things thrown in there. We were down to tying the straps into loops and ratcheting them down as tight as we could by that point.

We stopped somewhere at a Tractor Supply and bought another chain and binder, which turned out to be a very lucky thing. In Dallas the temperature began to drop and the rain started. By the time we made it out into the open plains of west Texas it was twenty-seven degrees and snowing. The overpasses were iced over and we were just sliding across them trying to make it to the next town to find someplace to stop without wrecking. We didn't.

I was driving crossing an overpass just outside of Sweetwater. It swept to the right, we went straight. I'm not sure how long we were airborne. It seemed like a pretty long time. Long enough for me to look over at Jackson and say "Looks bad." Then all kinds of stuff started happening real fast.

We hit the ground, hard. A great big highway sign was coming at us then the truck hit its pole and it slammed down on top of us, smashing down the roof and the top of the windshield. Sparkly little bits of glass rained down everywhere. It would have been kind of festive if not for the circumstances, and the fact that they were stabbing into our faces and hands. We ran up the embankment and across the oncoming lanes then slammed against the guardrail and came to rest looking up an ice-slicked hill, hoping not to see any vehicles coming our way.

I tried to turn to check out the trailer and bus but couldn't. Somebody was shoving a red-hot poker into my upper spine every time I tried to turn my head.

"Jack I can't see, is the bus still there?" I asked.

"Damn, everything's still hooked up, it doesn't even look like its moved," he answered.

"We've got to get out of here," I said.

I shifted the truck into four-wheel low and pulled away from the rail then started up the oncoming lane.

"What are you doing?" Jack asked incredulously as I started to turn off the roadway and down the shoulder when we got past the guardrail.

"If a truck comes over that hill, we're dead." I answered. We half drove half skidded down the bank, drove over a fence, and got onto the access road. The only thing I could think of to do was to keep crippling along the access road for the fourteen miles into Sweetwater, and call the police. We spent two days in a Holiday Inn Express. It didn't really help. I didn't feel all that much smarter.

All we could do was wait to get a break in the weather. Watching the local forecasts on TV we saw that if we could get a hundred miles south the temperature was in the forties. So we got back on the interstate, the top of the windshield splinted with duct tape and looking out through the spider-webbed glass, we drove on at fifteen to twenty miles per hour headed for California.

We passed thirty-one wrecked tractor-trailers and an overturned salt truck in the next seventy-five miles. We later learned eight people had died on that stretch of road in that storm.

The rest of the trip wasn't uneventful either, there was dense fog on I-10, and a windstorm that blew over four tractor-trailers between Phoenix and Los Angeles, but all that kind of seemed like a breeze by that point.

We can stop here, but the story didn't.

In Los Angeles the electrical problems returned, we later found out that they were the result of a failure to connect the ground wire when the engine was replaced, and the bus died repeatedly leaving us stranded on the 110, the 101, and the 210 freeways with traffic zipping around us. After that, all shooting on the bus was done with it <u>on</u> the flatbed.

I returned from Los Angeles and had x-rays made of my spine, which showed that what I had diagnosed as a disc problem was in actuality a compression fracture of the T3 vertebrae. When my wife found out she threatened to break my neck.

The One About the Warthogs

I know that in a previous story I've already talked ad nauseum about my failure to see the inherent dangers that certain animals pose as a result of a childhood filled with a few too many cartoons. Specifically, the trouble it almost got me into with a pair of young lions. Several of you, if you read the previous story, are probably thinking that you're going to come through this written page and strangle me to death with your bare hands if I bring up the word anthropomorphism or refer to Disney in any form what so ever. So, I won't. Well I already did, but that was just to tell you that I wasn't going to.

But you have to admit that with some animals it's pretty easy to see the folly of thinking of wild things as inherently sweet and friendly. As I said before sharks are a wonderful example of that. Hammerheads scare me to death personally, because I can never tell where they're looking. In my opinion, Dorothy, the Scarecrow, and the Tin Man hit the high points fairly well when it comes to what we should obviously be afraid of, "Lions and tigers and bears. Oh my."

It gets a little harder to stay objective, however, when you get to know the animals in question on a personal level. Now, I will admit that when I was in Namibia I never completely relaxed with Maggie, the cheetah. She was a wonderful day to day companion, that we hand fed, scratched behind the ears and talked to, and she was terribly sweet, licking you with her sandpaper tongue and purring in a gravely way that almost sounded like a growl. But, once you saw her go after the yard dogs if they happened to get too close something she was eating, you couldn't really let go of that image.

A cheetah up close is lightning quick, and can silently go from calm placidity to a whirling vortex of teeth and claws in an instant. That she could possibly go from a purring big kitty cat, to slicing you into confetti just as quickly was never too far from your mind. As a result of Maggie's mercurial transformations, the dogs tended to be skittish and, to some extent, so was I.

Ruthie, the pet warthog, on the other hand, looked just like a miniature version of Pumba and would trot right up to you, head up and tail straight as a flagpole, to nuzzle against your leg. I saw her as my personal pet for our visit to Africa. With her sunny disposition and obvious happiness to get any morsel of food she was offered, it was hard to see her as anything else.

A few days after my encounter with the lions at the fence, I was in back of the garage and Ruthie came trotting over to me. I can remember thinking to myself, maybe we've been feeding her a little bit too much. She's growing like a weed. I reached down to scratch her ear and she whirled more abruptly than usual bashing into my leg and trotting off. When I walked on up to the house, to wash-up for lunch, Fritz, the father in our father-son team of professional hunters, looked at me curiously.

"What were you doing with that pig?" He asked, in his thick Boor accent.

"Scratching its ears," I replied.

"Well, don't do it to the wild ones any more, they'll take the jewels right out from between your legs, and leave you wondering what's happened." He warned.

"Wild ones? I thought that was Ruthie." I sputtered.

"Ruthie? What, are you blind boy? That pigs more than twice her size. They're getting in through the gap in the fence. Give 'em some space and don't box 'em up and you'll be fine, but don't go about trying to pat on them, for heaven's sake."

I spent most of lunch picturing myself with a warthog devouring a personally cherished part of my anatomy. Fritz spent lunch telling us about the hunter that almost bled to death, and ended up requiring seventy-five stitches, when a long tusked, boar warter darted out of the brush and sliced him from knee to groin with a razor sharp lower tusk.

"It's the lower tusk that you have to watch." He explained, "The upper tusk looks bigger, but it's the sheath, it's the bottom tusk that does the cutting."

At this point I have to admit that I may have altered the exact nature and language of some of the exchanges that have and will take place in this story. With Fritz's accent, age and demeanor the language he used seemed perfectly appropriate at the time, but as with much creative profanity, it kind of suffers in transcription. Since we're trying to keep this suitable for a general audience, you'll have to make do with what's written and use your imagination to provide specific inflection from here on out.

On our hunt later that afternoon, I was the number two hunter. So it was, walking along, tongue stuck to the roof of your mouth, taking pictures, and trying to stay out of the way while your partner hunted. When we got home a curious thing happened, my boot wouldn't come off of my foot, I pulled and pulled, but except for a dull pain in the middle of my foot nothing happened.

I'm a physician, I know about things. Shoes don't just get stuck on people's feet. So, I started to examine the boot to try and figure out what was holding it in place. Feeling along just below the laces I found the tip of a thorn poking up through the leather. I twisted my foot over and there, embedded in the sole of my boot, was the thorns base.

I'd gotten my tetanus booster before I left the U.S. so that wasn't a problem. But I still had to get the boot off my foot. A set of Leatherman pliers I carry with me wherever I hunt and a sharp jerk, and the problem was solved. I held the bloody thorn and looked at it. So sharp that it had pierced boot and foot when I jumped off of the truck, and I never even felt it.

The next morning, my foot was sore and swollen. I couldn't walk much because my boot was too tight. So, we sat in a blind at a water hole, with a camera, marveling at the diverse collection of birds and animals that inhabit the central plateau of Namibia. By lunch I had seen more species of animals and birds than you could in a year anywhere outside of Africa. With a camera full of pictures, we headed home for lunch and a nap. I'd decided not to hunt that evening either, to give my foot a little more time to recover.

As we got out of the truck I grabbed my rifle. I'd left it in the truck all morning. It had been soaked by the dew then covered with the fine powder of red dust that covers everything in that place. I knew I needed to wipe it down with a little gun oil to keep the bolt from binding, so I unloaded it and carried it back to the garage, where I slept in a room between Fritz and the cook.

I chose to sleep in the garage instead of the picturesque thatched walled guest cabins for a purely practical reason, its walls were made of tin instead of thatch, less worries about lizards, snakes, and spiders. Oh, you still had to be sure to dump your shoes out in the morning, but at least they weren't jumping down on your face in the middle of the night. It was one of those things you hear from some old hunter, and file away in the back of your brain somewhere, as a lesson you may not need to learn first-hand. Unfortunately, for them, it was a lesson that my two fellow travelers from Mississippi learned the hard way.

As I approached the door Fritz was standing there looking at it.

"You didn't leave the door open this morning, did you?" he asked.

"Nope," I said. "I came out before you did, remember."

"Damned cook." He muttered to himself.

I walked into the small bedroom, closed the door behind me, and tossed the rifle onto the spare bed.

That's when all hell broke loose.

Three adult warthogs darted out from under the bed. I screamed like a girl and jumped onto the other bed, and five or six warthogs ran out from under that bed to join the other three, which were now running laps around and around the room. I jumped over to the bed with the rifle, startling the already upset pigs even more, and started fumbling in my pocket for shells. Luckily, common sense overcame me before I found any. I was in a small room with a cement floor, and tin walls. If I fired a gun in there somebody, and probably not a pig, was going to get hurt. I jumped back to the first bed keeping the rifle with me to use as a club and tried to reach the door, too far. So I tried to push it open with the barrel of the rifle. The pigs, un-use to people jumping and swinging guns around them, started so vocalize, in huffing squeals, snap at each other, and make little rushes at the bed I was on.

This was not good, and I could tell that my nap was going to be ruined if I didn't get some help in resolving this issue fairly quickly. I did the only thing I could think of, I started hollering at the top of my lungs for Fritz. When he opened the door to see what I was hollering about, he was almost bowled over, as three of the warters made their escape. The rest ran back under the beds.

"What in the bloody hell are you doing in there?" He shouted startled.

"I'm jumping from bed to bed. What in the hell does it look like I'm doing in here?"

"But, why are the pigs in there, and why did you throw your clothes at them?" he asked, truly puzzled.

"That would be a good question, and no I didn't throw my clothes at them. I guess they were trying to get the gum and candy I had in my suitcase." I replied.

"Well you need to get 'em out of there."

"You're the professional hunter, how do you suggest I do that?" I inquired.

"Well, for starters I wouldn't get off of the bed."

"I don't think that's something you're going to have to worry about." I said looking down to see glimpses of snouts and tails under the bed across the room.

"Second thing, put down the gun." He ordered.

"Like hell I will." I countered.

"Look, I'll throw you a broom. You drop the rifle, and if you don't ruin the scope entirely, we're going to spend all day tomorrow trying to re-sight-in your rifle." He explained patiently.

No one sights in a .416 for fun, so I laid it gently on the bed.

"Toss me the broom." I capitulated.

The next thirty minutes was spent jumping from bed to bed, poking the porkers out from under one bed only to have them run under the other, it took us that long to figure out that the pigs were afraid of Fritz who remained watching in the doorway.

"Okay, run in here and jump on this other bed." I suggested, "Then you can keep them from getting under the bed you're on when I get them out from under this bed."

"I have a better idea," he replied.

Through the doorway I could see him throwing a pail of corn down in the courtyard, and true to form Ruthie appeared and started to munch away. I suppose pigs, like people, most want whatever it is that other pigs have got. So, one by one, the remaining porkers scooted out the door and set about eating the corn. When the last one was gone I hopped to the other bed and looked back just to be sure there weren't any stragglers before I darted to the door and slammed it shut.

And that, my friends was the end of the one about the warthogs, or so

I thought...

When I re-entered the United States, the customs officials in Miami stopped me. A dog sniffed at my clothing and then my suitcase, alerting everyone in a fifty-yard radius. One of the officials approached me briskly and said, "We're going to need to go through all of your luggage."

"Why?" I asked. "Is there a problem?"

"Well, the dog's smelled something. We have to be sure that you aren't transporting any contraband." She explained.

"What kind of contraband?" I asked, beginning to get concerned.

"This dog is trained to detect meat," she said. "We have reason to believe that you may be trying to smuggle illegal meat into the United States."

And you know? For a minute there, when they first opened up that suitcase, I was kind of afraid that I was.

The End of the World

We've all heard of the old Chinese curse, "May you live in interesting times." Well unfortunately, if you subscribe to the same point of view as cursing Chinamen, we do. Contrary to popular belief, not all of the interesting stuff that's happening in the world we inhabit is political, economic, or concerned with the best way to lose weight. There have been some really exciting things happening in the area of basic and theoretical physics lately. Most of us would probably have missed it, except for a couple of headlines that screamed out.

PHYSICS EXPERIMENT MAY LEAD TO END OF WORLD

That's one of the unfortunate things about basic physics research. A lot of times, because the stuff we're interested in has to do with the kind of stuff that devours whole solar systems, there's this teeny tiny chance we might accidentally...blow up the whole planet.
Now obviously that's a bad thing, and one of the types of things we should probably try to avoid at all costs. Its not that I'm against progress or anything, it's just that, for mankind, we have this peculiar attachment to maintaining our planet. Because...well I guess the best reason is...

IT'S THE ONLY ONE WE HAVE

For most of the three to four hundred thousand years there have been people walking around on the earth, our planet has really been the only universe we knew anything about. Even when the only things we knew anything about was the stuff right around us, there was still plenty of stuff to be afraid of. Saber-tooth tigers, floods, and wars are a few of the things that spring immediately to mind.

Then a couple of hundred years ago we found out that we might not be the exact center of the universe. The church didn't like this idea that much and did their best to try and get folks to just forget about all that astronomy stuff. But it just hung around, and in the process gave us a whole bunch of new things to worry about. Like asteroids, comets, and other things that might fly out of the sky and squish us.

In the last couple of decades we've learned that it's even worse than we thought. We actually live in one of a whole bunch of swirling galaxies, in a gigantic universe full of scary stuff. We didn't even want to think of what a supernova or black hole could do to our little blue ball of a planet, so we all decided we would just forget all about science and just stick to self-help books and weight loss diets from now on. It seemed like the more stuff we knew about, the more stuff there was that could theoretically annihilate us.

The expansion of human knowledge, in other words, had not been really all that comforting. There's also the problem that while we were learning stuff we also managed to make a few mistakes. Well, mistakes may not be the right word, but we did have a few unintended consequences. Can the world really be any more over than it is for the amazing number of native populations decimated by smallpox, syphilis, and tuberculosis spread by well meaning explorers? We weren't planning to kill anybody. We were just trying to find out more about the world we live in.

I can hear you saying, "That's ancient history. We're not like that anymore. We know what we're doing now."

No we don't. Hell, we weren't completely sure when we set off the first "H-bomb" that it wouldn't set off a chain reaction that would light up all of the hydrogen floating around our little planetary home. We didn't think it would and it didn't, but who knew? Certainly, not the guys that did it.

Which brings us back to the story of the scary headlines. The European Center for Nuclear Research is a scientific cooperative that's been around a year longer than I have. It was founded in 1954 as one of Europe's first joint ventures, and has contributed some of the most important fundamental scientific observations of the last half-century. They've had access to the most advanced scientific instruments available at any given time. But what they are doing is of an order of magnitude more complex than anything we've seen before. The headlines referred to the approaching power-on for a complex scientific device called the Large Hadron Collider.

Because I have a background in physics the subject was one that was brought up to me in conversations several times recently. Usually along the lines of, "Do you think when they turn that big collider on, over there in Europe, it's going to be the end of the world?" My answer was a not very reassuring, "I guess it could."

The chances of the accelerated protons or lead ions that scientists were planning to send racing around the new thirteen-mile nuclear racetrack they'd built three-hundred feet below the ground over on the Franco-Swiss border, forming a black-hole that doesn't dissipate, or an uncontrolled annihilation reaction due to anti-matter generation was less than one in fifty-million.

The good news, if you believe in string theory, is that even if it happened, we may end up in one of the other ten, twenty, or hundred other dimensions we aren't able to see, but that have to be there for the universe to work right.

I started thinking about all of this because of those great big headlines. They wrote the headlines because of a lawsuit. I'm sure there have been other lawsuits filed to stop scientific experiments, but this is the first time I've ever heard of one being filed because the folks bringing it were afraid that the experiment was going to blow up the planet.

A group of concerned citizens tried to stop them from turning on the Large Hadron Collider and block the construction of any other "Super-Colliders" in the future. Now a super-collider is just great big donut shaped machine that gets all of the air sucked out of it, to make a vacuum, then it gets cooled down to $-273°$ C which is designated as $0°$ on the Kelvin scale. That, by itself takes about three months. Once we have an absolute vacuum at $0°$ K we can shoot some charged particles in there and use magnetic fields to speed them up as fast as we can, then slam them into a dense metalallic target, and see what happens.

Of course there are a few risks like: forming a black-hole that doesn't dissipate or maybe even expands to swallow us and our solar system and probably a few of our neighboring stars all up. If that doesn't happen there's still the chance of an uncontrolled annihilation reaction secondary to anti-matter generation that sets up a chain reaction and turns all the mass on earth to pure energy. And if neither of those things kill us, there's yet a third risk called a strangelet phenomenon and I don't even know what that would look like.

Well the clock ticked on.

Lucky for science the concerned citizens failed. The accelerated nuclei took their first trip around that thirteen mile test track, and guess what? We're still here. No black holes, nothing. The particles just cut a hole in the wall, and tore everything up.

Still we have to feel kind of lucky that we didn't all wake up dead that Wednesday morning, because even if the odds were one in fifty million of something bad happening, if you're the one, it's still statistically significant for you.

Anyway, what I'm getting at is, all of this uproar about the end of the world reminded me of a story I read by Ray Bradbury back in high school. The story was about a family that knew that the world was going to end that night.

As a teen-ager, the ideas you have about what you would do if the world was going to end tend to center on sex, drugs, and alcohol, maybe, a really fast car. I think that's why that story stayed in my mind all these years. I knew what I'd want to do if the world was going to end, but the family in this story didn't do any of those things.

They just did all of the things that they did every other night. They ate their dinner, read some stories to their kids, put the kids to bed, kissed them goodnight, and went to sleep. As a teen-ager, the story was incomprehensible, the idea of doing nothing different, of just kissing each other good-night and going to sleep seemed almost overwhelmingly strange, but the more you thought about it, the more it made sense. That's an example of Bradbury's genius.

Now that I'm a parent it makes even more sense. You start to think about it in terms of your own life as a parent, and how you feel about your children. Not all of the time, but how you'd feel about them if you thought they were going to be dead in the morning.

So probably, the parents would be a lot nicer than usual. No one screaming, "Get to bed!" or "Don't you know tomorrow's a school day?" The mom probably made a nice dinner, one everybody liked. It would be all sweet and nice.

Dad would say, "Homework...schmomework, lets just forget about that stupid math and pop a little popcorn tonight."

I have this nagging feeling though that, for some reason, it wouldn't be like that at my house, but maybe it would. We didn't lie awake waiting for them to light off the "Super-Collider". We just went to bed and went to sleep, just like the people in the story. It was easy for us. Nobody in my house except for me had ever heard of the Super-Collider.

But, what would we do if we <u>knew</u> the world was going to end. That's hard to say. What are you going to do? Drive all over the place trying to get off the earth, or out of our solar system? It's not like any of us have some space ark built out in the back yard, and it's not like we're going to build one. We wouldn't know a cubit if it bit us on the foot.

So what would we do? What did the people in the story do?

"Honey, did you read the paper this evening?"

"Yeah, did you read that thing about the end of the world?"

"That sure is strange isn't it, a black hole...now why would a black hole want to eat our section of the galaxy."

"I don't know, but they say it's supposed to get here about three in the morning."

What do you do then? I imagined a conversation with my own wife.

"Well what do you want to do tonight?"

"We ought to do something. It's the last night on earth?"

"Yeah, that's a lot bigger than New Years."

"We could order a bunch of things on the internet on our charge cards."

"Why would we want to do that?"

"Well, it's not like we're ever going to have to pay for all the stuff we order. So it's like getting it for free," she'd answered.

"But, you're never going to get it either." I'd say.

"But you'd know you bought it."

"Maybe I could get on e-bay and buy a bunch of Ferraris."

"But why would you want to do that?"

"I've always wanted a Ferrari, maybe I'll buy five, one of every model."

"Ferrari has five models. Who do they sell them to?"

"Well I counted the convertibles…"

"Why would you want five Ferraris?"

"Just for the sake of winning the auctions," I'd explain. "I can say to myself. 'See, I got every one of them.'"

"I'm not sure e-bay's such a good idea."

"You wanted to order stuff on the credit cards."

"But, if everybody knows the world is going to end tomorrow, everyone's going to bid like there's no tomorrow. BECAUSE THERE'S NO TOMORROW!"

"So what? That just means I'll have to work harder to get 'em. I'm only going to bid on stuff that ends tonight. Besides, I'm not really going to have to pay."

But what if you're wrong? What if it was all a giant mistake? The black hole took a left turn and ate Alpha Centauri or some other solar system instead of ours? We're just going to get a seven-year drought or something.

You wake up late for work the next morning. You didn't set the alarm clock. Why? You weren't supposed to wake up. Your whole family's running around like a bunch of chickens with their heads cut off. Mom's trying to get the kids ready for school.

"Who said you didn't have to do your Math homework?"

You're trying to get ready for work. The kids are wondering what in the heck's going on.

"Boy, they were so nice last night. Now they're hollering like crazy. Dad cussed a blue streak because he forgot to put the garbage out last night (it wasn't supposed to be there in the morning)."

Then you remember the five Ferraris, the ones you were bidding against all the other poor saps that didn't think the world was going to be here this morning either. What was the final bid? Thirty-four trillion apiece?

"Oh crap," you exclaim, watching the neighbor shoving his three kids still in their pajamas into his Suburban. "I put that on the American Express, the one with no limit."

Now that's the end of the world.

I don't know how these things get into my head, but I'm happy to pass them on.

Caught

The black limousine slowed and came to a stop a block away from the entrance of the only luxury resort in Uzbekistan. I looked out of the window at the road, and then across the back seat at my wife and daughter. I knew why I was here. I had to meet a man who had recovered a set of microfiche that detailed the assembly and disassembly of a W-79 Mod 1 warhead. As far as nuclear weapons went, it wasn't much, about a half of a kiloton. But this one had neutron capabilities. The fiche had to be retrieved. There were no options. There was no question. I knew what I had to do, I'd done it before in Egypt. The only thing bothering me was: Why were my wife and daughter here? What could have possessed me to bring them on something like this?

I got out of the car on the street side when I saw a man in a grey coat approach the vehicle. He motioned me to the trunk, raised it to provide cover, and handed me a briefcase.

"Your papers, passports, money, and the package are all in this. What you need is sewed into the lining," he said with no trace of an accent.

"Anything else?" I asked

"This," he said handing me a tiny weapon. "It's fully automatic, a .17 caliber. It's a prototype."

I looked at the weapon and turned it over. A Springfield Armory cartouche was stamped on its side.

"Don't use it unless you have to but don't hesitate if you need to," he instructed. "I'll take you to your room."

He got into the front of the limo and we pulled to the door. When the doorman opened the back, I slid across the seat to follow my family. As I started to get out the contact offered his hand.

"Let me help you," he said taking the briefcase and handing it to my wife. I got out of the car and put my arm around my daughter's shoulders to shield her from the blast of cold wind. Walking into the lobby a baggage cart hit me and I stumbled. Through the hanging bags I saw the contact pushing my wife, the briefcase still in her hands into an elevator. I grabbed my daughter's hand and started around the cart. I saw panic in my wife's face as the elevator doors closed.

I looked around quickly, this wasn't a main elevator bank, there were no floors numbered above the doors. I had no idea where they were going. I started for the stairs to the Mezzanine, but stopped cold when I saw two government people checking passports. I looked across the lobby and spotted two more checking everyone as they entered the main elevators.

How did I let this happen? I had no papers, no passports, no microfiche, and no wife. On top of all that my daughter was right beside me. Anything that went wrong would put her at risk. I could only imagine how pleased the Uzbekistani police were going to be with a guy with no passport, no papers, and carrying an automatic weapon with an identifiable U.S. manufacturer.

I walked down a long hallway labeled "spa" in English, Japanese, and Cyrillic. As I passed a waste container I dropped the weapon wrapped in my daughter's scarf into it. Suddenly a large man in a plaid sport coat and cowboy boots was coming across the hallway with his hand extended and a big smile on his face.

"Hey, doc," he said from fifty feet away.

No one here knew I was a doctor. I dropped a T-handle blade from its sheath on my wrist down into my right hand, and kept the blade up so that it was invisible.

I'll spin him and take out the left kidney as I go around. I can't let him reach the kid, I thought.

"Hey doc, remember me. It's Brad Dorland from Laurel. You cured my prostate cancer six years ago. I'll never forget that face. What in the hell are you doing here in Uzbekistan?" He continued.

I dumped the knife into my coat pocket as I brought my hand around to shake his. "Hey Mr. Dorland. I guess you're still in the oil business?" I said, remembering.

"Yep, that's why I'm here, I've got to re-negotiate these leases every time these guys change governments. Hell, I know people in Mississippi that don't change clothes as fast as these guys change leaders. But what's a cancer doctor doing over here?"

"I'm supposed to be giving a lecture on cervical cancer tomorrow, but I'll be damned if I know if I'm going to make it." I answered glumly.

"What's wrong doc?" He asked.

"I forgot my passport up in my room, I've got my daughter here with me, and those government goons are checking everybody going up and down into the building. I don't know what to do." I explained, almost telling the truth.

"I can get you up there, but we have to go through the sauna. You're going to have to cover that young ladies eyes though; those guys in there are naked as jaybirds….."

BUZZZ ZZZZ ZZZZ BUZZZZ ZZZ ZZZ ZZZ BUZZZ ZZZZ ZZZZ BUZZZ ZZZ ZZZ

I smacked the sleep button and tried to go back to sleep to see how things turned out, but it was no use. Charlene had heard it and she and her pack of aggravating dogs descended on the bedroom.

"Maddie has a field trip, so you're going to have to pick up Allison at basketball practice…"

I listened but I wasn't hearing, I need to figure out what had happened in Uzbekistan. Was Charlene okay? I think Allison was the daughter in the dream, but it was starting to fade and I wasn't sure anymore.

I was caught, caught in that area between dreams and reality. Where you know what's real, but you can't let go of what you know isn't. It's like dreaming you had a fight with your wife and waking up mad at her. You know it's unreasonable, but you can't help it.

I lumbered down the steps in my robe and slippers to get my coffee.

How stupid could I have been? I should have known it was a set-up when I saw the cartouche on the gun. Nobody on an op uses a marked gun, especially not a prototype. Why would they have even given me a prototype? You would have wanted a throw away.

I finished my coffee and got into the shower.

I never saw the microfiche. How did I even know they were there? How would they have possibly gotten to Uzbekistan?

I got dressed and got into my car.

I think my wife was in on it. She wouldn't have put her own child in danger, would she? I don't think she was really panicked at all? Sure she has blonde hair and blue eyes, but she could have been recruited in Sweden couldn't she. Besides, what did I really know about her. We'd only been married seventeen years.

It was hard to concentrate on my first consult, but then, I focused. This person's real life was in my hands, and they deserved my undivided, my full attention. By lunchtime the dream was gone.

That isn't always the case though. Two days later I was seeing a follow-up patient that I had treated for a brain tumor a year earlier. His scans were fine, no masses, no enhancement, and no hydrocephalus.

"How are you doing?" I asked going in the door.

"How's the scan say I'm doing?" he countered.

"If you're as good as the scans say you are, you can get your butt right on out of here, cause I don't have a bunch of time to waste on somebody that doesn't have anything wrong with them." I said smiling.

"That's great. I was sure you were going to find something," he said, clearly relieved.

"Why do you say that? Have you been having headaches?" I asked.

"No, no nothing like that. It's my arms."

"What's wrong with your arms? Are they numb…weak?" I continued.

"Nah, they feel like I dipped them in fiberglass. They itch all the time." He said rolling up his sleeves and extending his forearms.

His arms were excoriated and red. The skin was dry. But, there was no clear rash.

"You got dry skin, have you been putting anything on them."

"Yeah, I have to, I forgot to put it on when I got out of the shower this morning,"

"When did this start? Was it after they gave you the contrast for the scans?" I thought I had the answer.

"I can tell you just when it started. It started when I had that dream." He explained.

"What dream?"

"See, I dreamed my arms was all in this poison oak. I was shucking these little beans out, and there was poison oak everywhere, it was all up against me. I woke up just scratching my arms like crazy. Do you think it's all in my head? I thought maybe it was the tumor making me think this way, but you said the scans were good."

"I think it started off in your head. You woke up scratching, your skin was dry, the scratching caused your body to release histamines and so you itched more. The more you scratched the more you itched. It's kind of a vicious cycle. Let's try some anti-histamines and see if it goes away."

"Well, I guess that seems like a good idea." He said, then his face clouded and he continued. "My arms itching is part of it, but that's not what's really worrying me. What's bothering me is <u>why</u> my arms is itching. That's what's got me puzzled."

"Remember what I said about the histamine release…"

"I know what you said. But, that's not what's funny about it. You know what the funny thing about all this is?"

"No, what?" I asked.

"I'm not even allergic to poison oak."

Both stories are true, that shows the power of dreams.

Author's Note: This is an experimental bit of interactive literature I'm throwing in. The Ghost was originally a column by itself, as was a hybrid piece that combined The Continuation and The Thomasine Confluence, but I've included the entirety of the expansions, so that they are seen in context to one another. If you don't like them or they get tedious for you just skip on over to Eavesdropping. I put it next as a treat. Wait, wait, wait…Get back here! You can't just go straight there, at least try to read this one. Who knows, it may be one of your favorites?

The Ghost and the Book Wright Expansions

1.)   The Ghost

I don't know much about ghost stories. I don't like reading them 'cause my life is scary enough as it is. You want to scare me you can hold the ghosts and tell me about a woman and her two daughters loose in Bergdorf's with my credit card, now that's what scares the hell out of me. As far as trying to tell one, I was never any good at 'em. I usually messed up the scary part, and everybody'd laugh when they were supposed to be hollering and screaming. Although that happens about a lot of stuff, for me, the laughing part not the hollering and screaming. I guess it's just the way I say things.

I remember once when I was just going into radiation oncology and was still doing a lot of work at the Children's Hospital of the Kings Daughter. I was trying to tell a friend who I'd deployed with on dive jobs around the world about how it was making me feel. How I was running a lot better now because I wasn't running through woods imagining getting away from Russians or Arabs or whatever, I was running down the streets of Virginia Beach trying to get away from the eyes of the dead children I'd taken care of.

His response wasn't that helpful in trying to help me find a way to deal with the way I was feeling about stuff. He cracked up and said, "Man you should do stand-up. This stuff is hilarious."

I changed the subject.

So if you're hoping for a scary ghost story save yourself the trouble and bail out now, 'cause that's not what this is going to be. Anyway, Barry Hannah died this month. He was the kind of author that took chances, sometimes too many, but he was a good writer, for it and despite it too. He died up in Oxford where he taught creative writing, but I never knew him there. He was born here in the town where I live, Meridian Mississippi, but I never knew him here either. I went to the University of Alabama. When I was there we won the national championship twice, Bear Bryant was our coach, Sela Ward was one of our cheerleader, and Barry Hannah was a drunken whirlwind, shooting arrows through folks houses, stealing motorcycles, and teaching in the English Department. That's when I was aware of his existence.

I wasn't the kind to get too impressed with a wild ass literature professor back then, I was in the honors English program and was studying Southern Literature because I liked it, but I was a pre-med major and all I gave a shit about was Biochemistry, and Physics, and Advanced Analytic Spectroscopic technique. My one stab at writing was a research paper on "The Clinical and Laboratory Characteristics of Macroamylasemia" a clinical syndrome where your amylase molecules are too big, with large redundant sections, so it doesn't get excreted normally and you get high serum amylase levels. I'm pretty sure Barry wouldn't have seen it favorably, as it didn't take a lot of chances with the English language. Anyway, <u>Airships</u> had just come out, and one of the big stories that drew a lot of local ire was <u>Constant Pain in Tuscaloosa</u>. The constant pain had ended up with him in Bryce Hospital, the local inpatient psychiatric unit, for alcoholism. Which explains some things later in the story.

Now this morning was a rodeo Saturday at Casa Charlo (that's the name we gave our new house, the last one was called The Monkey House because of all of the kids who lived in it with us). We were up a 5:45 am to get ready, get everything together; horses, trailers, trucks, etcetera so the girls could drive across the state to ride horses around stuff in a dirt pen somewhere else instead of here. I wasn't going, so after I took them to breakfast and the barn and watched them drive away in a pick-up with a gooseneck horse trailer on the back I got to go home and go back to bed for another hour or so.

That's when Barry showed up. Which was kind of disconcerting, because I'd known about him being dead for about a week or so. Anyway, I was lying there asleep and there he was, his hair was even still dark, no gray in it yet, although he died with a bunch of gray hair. He was leaning over the bed and shouting down into my face, like he was famous for doing in class all those years ago.

"Tom...Tom...listen to me now Tom." My names not Tom, but I figured it was the alcohol talking. "...just listen. You're never going to be a real writer if you keep yourself all bottled up in your own life. You got to let go. You just got to let go and see what in the hell happens. Let your characters run their own lives. Stop getting in the middle of it. You gonna be dead soon enough, just like me. Write something worth leaving before you go Tom. God damn it, write something worth leaving."

It never occurred to me that he might of gotten the wrong address, somehow I knew he was talking to me, he just had the wrong name, which wasn't unusual back then either.

"So what is it you're trying to tell me to do, man?" I asked, still in college, I suppose.

"When opportunity knocks, you open the door Tom. Open the fuckin' door."

In the dream, I guess, I heard the doorbell ring and I was confused. Barry was gone and I didn't know if the doorbell had really rung or not. The dogs weren't barking. That was a sign that it was just in the dream, but I couldn't just lay there. I got up and put on my robe and went from door to door and I didn't see anybody out there. Opportunity had not knocked.

I tried to figure it all out, but it didn't make sense. I poured a cup of coffee and sat down at my desk and rewrote the ending of <u>The Hard Times</u>, the novel I was editing, and I wrote well, which is always a nice thing. It was raining outside, the coffee was still warm, and I knew that while opportunity knocks and is gone, inspiration's the one that takes the time to ring the bell.

2.) The Continuation

When I posted my little story *The Ghost* on my blog it produced an interesting set of responses, which I shall post here, via the magic of cut and paste, the names have been changed to protect the innocent.

Sis: Enjoyed the blog, Tom. Glad you answered when opportunity rang the bell"

Frank: "Tom, are you sure it wasn't UPS...they ring once and run. And, we went to RMH for the Cardiac Unit's 2 year anniversary this afternoon. Shook hands with my Surgeon, his PA, nurses etc., who remembered me well.....when leaving, the Surgeon said "nice seeing you again - you look great, Tom".... When they made my name tag....they put Thomas (my middle name) instead of Frank....very - very spooky if you ask me....Tom........VERY SPOOKY.....!!!!"

Me: "the world is a spooky place maybe he was in the wrong place"

Frank: "Which Tom was in the wrong place?"

Ms CGS: "or maybe the surgeon is a closet writer/blogger/prf. of English?"

Me: "Frank, since you're the only Tom here, I think the ghost was a bit south of where he intended to be."

Frank: "But, you see, I'm NOT the only Tom here...you have a Tom there....You are just as much of a Tom as I am....mistaken identity?"

Ms CGS: "can I play? I'll be Tom the Editor.

Frank: "hmmm.....I think there are 2 impostors...will the REAL Tom please stand up.....(the quickest solution)."

Frank: "OMG...we all stood up at the same time...back to square one.

3.) The Thomasine Confluence

I was planning to answer CGS with a suggestion that if we were going to cast an attractive woman as Tom the editor, that she would have to be comfortable being a domin-ed-trix , you know, an editor that was only able to enjoy editing when she could dress up in clothes from Versace and edit writers really, really hard. But then something struck me. It was both the tone and the content of those final two posts which led me to the conclusion that there was something larger going on here. So that meant it was time for me to get in gear and look into it, in the way only a piercing mind such as mine can possibly do it. It was time for some...tat da da daaaaaah.....(wait on it)......RESEARCH.

Now research is always a good answer when you have a vexing problem or coincidence to investigate, the problem becomes how, and what to research? Clearly, this doesn't appear to be a religious problem, although the bible is replete with examples of Thomas's who play a prominent role in Biblical history, and there is always the possibility that we have all been simultaneously, because of our natural tendencies to scoff, and distrust been transformed into visages of the Thomas who doubted Jesus' resurrection, but after due consideration and running a few preliminary mathematical equations, I rejected this as the explanation. Although those of you that want to accept this as the answer on faith alone are welcome to do so.

Biology was another consideration, and I had to rule out the possibility that some genetic sequence that we all possess in common is the root of our mutual Thomasine misidentification. So, I went out to the garage and fired up my DNA sequencer, and used a vacuum on my screen to suck DNA samples from the keyboards of each of your computers, by visiting your Facebook profile, and using direct screen-to-screen transport to shove the vacuum nozzle against your keyboard. I hope you don't mind the intrusion. (Frank- I'm sorry about the mess. I pushed the blow button by mistake, but I changed the bag right after that. So the second time things went a lot better.)

I looked at the recovered DNA, and yes almost ninty-percent of our

DNA sequences are similar, but eighty-five percent of our DNA sequences match those of an earthworm, so I wasn't able to draw any firm scientific conclusions from that. And while I don't profess to speak fluent earthworm, I am unaware of any earthworms that refer to one another as Tom at all, much less it having some identifiable locus in their genome, so I was able to exclude those common sequences from consideration. The five percent remaining that the three of us have in common with each other, but not with earthworms seems to code for stuff like arms and legs and a four chamber heart and things like that, and not for name specific identity. So I rejected biology.

The answer then I reasoned must come from the realm of physics, specifically I gravitated to the subject of String Theory, and because it is such a fluid field, I adjusted and tweaked physical principles, added two unknown dimensions to account for Thomasine movement, a term I have now created, and viola there was the answer implicit in the very underpinnings of the science.

We have only to look of the dual resonance model, first postulated by Veneziano in 1968 to see what is happening. In short, Veneziano observed that the s- and t-channel vibrations that occurred in meson scattering were of exactly the same amplitude, on further observation the exact phenomena was observed in N-particle amplitudes that gave us the idea of harmonic, opposing amplitudes like that occurs in a one-dimensional model of linear string vibration. Obviously what is happening to us is a exact but opposite reaction, modulated through time by the presence of the two unseen dimensions of the great Brucine Confluence that effected Monty Python in the same years that Veneziano was developing his resonance model, and is only showing up now. I propose that we try to quantify B- (for Brucine) and T- (for Thomasine) confluent amplitudes and sit back and wait on the guys in Stockholm to send us that Nobel Prize I knew I was going to get some day. I'll start working on the math.

4.) Discovery

Frank: ahhhh...but did you really?

MS CGS: Then there's "Tom, Tom, Piper's son, Stole a pig an' away he run; pig was eat, Tom was beat, Tom went runnin' down the street." (secret Mason-esque code for the potential perils of tracking the Holy Grail) Finally, the esoteric revealed!

Frank: Pig was yummy tho..........

Me: I had totally missed the secret society scenario, the code though may take us as far back as Thomas a' Beckett Archbishop of Canterbury from 1162 until his death in 1170.

Me: Now all we need is the secret ring.

Frank: I got one, but can't tell you or let you see it....it's a secret :-|

Me: The truth is that his real name was Gilbert Beket Jr. it must be some linkage to the Thomasine conversion of 1169 that caused Henry II to kill him the following year, and thus he became Saint Thomas to both the Catholics and the Protestants.

Frank: My ring has a video of that.....oops....shhhhh.

Me: Now if I can just tie this all into String Theory by adding a couple of more dimensions, we've got that little trinket from Stockholm sewn up.

MS CGS: Do you suppose Disney's "Thomasina," the cat heroine (re: the divine feminine) is Gilbert reincarnated? Her worst hairball was a visage not of Christ, but of her nemesis, Henry II's rat-fink advisor. She gagged when she spied the secret decoder ring in her daily ration of Cracker Jack.

Me: The screenplay for the film was originally written by two guys, Robert Westerby and Paul Gallico. But, it was based on the 1957 novel by

Gallico; Thomasina, the Cat Who Thought She Was God. ...

Me: What more proof could we possibly need, it also explains what Frank is when he drops that ring into that big wine goblet he's got, he's such a cat lover.

MS CGS: It's the Fisherman's Ring. Tom-Gilbert is the Pope!

Frank: Da*n Cats.....watch my decoder for the cat's 9th life.....

5.) Nobel

When I read what I have stretched out before you, I must admit, my blood ran cold. I came upon it on that fool Anderson's blog. He'll be the first one that I kill, I fear.

When the nomination first came before me I laughed. I have been a member of the Nobel Physics committee for seven years and this was the first time any one had paid so little regard to the Nobel protocol that they'd submitted their own work, work that had not even been finished, much less published, for official consideration. I knew right then that this Anderson must be either a fool or a genius. My job was to figure out which.

When I began to look through the submitted equations that were purported to prove the Thomasine Confluence theory, I was appalled. They lacked coherence and anywhere that they crashed they were buoyed by the insertion of an unseen universe or a temporal inversion to sustain them.

Officially I derided them, in public it was easy to show that they deserved no more consideration than the lint under my carpets for serious candidacy for the prize, but it took me to the blog, and it was when I read the comments that I knew they'd begun to see the clues.

My name is Ingateria Moelusteian, but everyone calls me Tom, and yes I am that Tom, the direct spiritual successor to the apostle Thomas, Saint Thomas, Thomas Jefferson, Tommy Smothers, and Tommy Chong. The Rightfully Ordained Brother Thomas of the Order of the Thomasine Monks. I am the guardian of the secret of cynical thoughts, the doubters of truth, God's own troublemakers. And now a small group of idiotic Americans had begun to post the secrets of our Order on the Internet.

My charge is clear, I must hunt them down one by one and eliminate them as a threat, by conversion to the true belief or transition to the inanimate.

6.) The Ring

Frank: "....(aka) Tom Was surfing the web (that's the information highway of the future), with his secret decoder ring, when he broke out in a cold sweat and yelled "OMG"!! He saw that Cracker Jack was NO LONGER putting the secret decoder rings in the boxes as prizes. That means that Frank (Tom) has the only one left. He also found out while surfing on the Anderson blog, that Inganteria Moelusteian wants the ring and has plans to 'inanimate' him to get it.....Thinking fast, Frank (Tom) quickly sold the secret decoder ring to a band of roaming gypsies roaming the Appalachian Mountains. Frank (Tom) then fled to the 'old country' where he will hide in the 'olcooedootdso' caves (known only to a few trusted minions) for the next 1,000 years. At that time he will retrieve the ring from the gypsies grave and again read the Anderson blog to see if it is safe for him to return to the general population."

Carl: "Tom Tom the piper runs 'n Scott had no wipes so some be stunned..."

MS CGS: "MY GOD, MAN, DON'T PAAAANICCC! Sick the Body Parinoid on this ingrate Inganteria. They'll devour principles held dear, then claim the ring was all their idea, after all. (Tom, embrace the Pope that is your true id.)"

Frank: "The ring is in safe hands, it has a 1,000 year curse on it....to be broken only by me....I MUST hide, paranoid cannot kill paranoid....it can only multiply! Inganteria is multiple paranoid.....run...hide..."

MS CGS: "Raiders of the Lost Ring, led by the intrepid but wily Jack Sparrow, intend to find you and that bejeweled metal circle. You can't hold for a century that freeze in Madame Troussaud's. Besides, we'd miss you, Mr. T. Take pride in your Tomness. If Obama can pass Health Care, you can face this fire!"

Frank: "'tis too late......the present and future has been written...in the 'olcooedootdso' caves, time is not time as you or I know it.....1,000 years is but.............mere weeks.......the fate of the secret decoder cannot and will not be changed."

7.) The Cavern

She'd grown up in the caverns. She was used to them. The cool velvet blackness did not frighten her. There was some comfort to it. As a constant temperature of 54° surrounded her she let herself adjust. The attack had been swift and sudden she'd never seen it coming. She was walking through the lobby with a newspaper and a cup of coffee when he grabbed her. What happened then was pure instinct. The fresh hot coffee had gone in his face. His hands came up to protect his eyes but it was too late. The scalding liquid seared his flesh and blistered his eyelids. The rolled newspaper stabbed straight forward into his groin and she was running. But She was already in the mouth of the cave when she heard the first sounds of his pursuit.

The sounds of her feet on the limestone steps, cut into the very mouth of the cave, sounded like thunder in her ears. She took comfort in that it because so would his.

"The ring!," he whispered harshly into her ear as he grabbed her. "I want the ring now..."

That was the only thing he said to her, before she turned and threw scalding liquid into his face. It wouldn't matter now if he could see her not, she thought as she reached the bottom of the grotto. She'd sat still and listened, listened as his footsteps came down those same stairs that she had just descended. It was only when she knew that he had reached the bottom beyond the reach of the light at the entrance that she threw the switch and threw them into utter and total darkness. It was a darkness deeper than any darkness and space because even in the outskirts of space some light from some distant source penetrates the blackness. Here there was none.

It was a funny thing, standing here in the pitch black, remembering how it was as a child. When she and her brothers and sisters have played in the caverns. Even in the dark, they had learned to feel one another. She wasn't sure how they did it. Maybe it was the feeling of the heat of another body passing by and the constant unvarying temperature of the underground environment. But sometime from somewhere she felt as a pastor in a dark. Leaving the uninitiated giving them faint sounds and echoes to follow. She took him to the edge of a drop off and stopped, waiting, silent, breathing as shallowly as she could. Even willing her heart to slow and beat in the control that only a lifetime of training can impart. Her thumb moved to the ring, and spun it on her finger as she waited. If she stood still at the base the stone column that she was leaning against he would pass her in the dark and in the passing would fall to his death. But would that solve her problem?

8.) Gypsies

Carl: "Wagner liked them."

Frank: "thought...........'RATZ, now I must come out of hiding....'
The caves are no longer safe.....He MUST get the ring from the Gypsies .... under the cover of darkness, Frank (Tom) moves out.....m-16 in hand......one target in mind...."

Gypsies, gypsies what in the hell had he been thinking of, trusting the ring to his cousins, now he was going to be tramping all over half of the state of West Virginia looking for that bunch of knuckleheads...and that's if they did what he told them to. He thought about Ms CGS, would he make it in time to save her, and was it even worth the trouble to try to. He'd had his suspicions about her as soon as he spoke to her over the phone. She'd know too much about the ring when they'd spoken, it was almost as if ... as if, she'd used the ring herself sometime, somewhere in the past. He hit a pothole, and heard the rifle bang against the back of the trucks cab, where he'd stored it behind the seat. Damn it, he hoped it stayed zeroed.

He should have just left it in the gun case until he got there. The problem was, that if he did run into Moelusteian unexpectedly, a gun in a case wasn't going to do him a whole lot of good.

Let him try his Swedish, paranoid, heresy here and see how much good it did him with an M-16 going off, up his butt. He turned up Das Valkyrie on his CD player. It wasn't Nibelung he was worried about, he had to find Willie and the Glimmer twins to get the ring back.

9.) Underground

Ms CGS: "The intensity of the moments, her breathlessness, the karst's vast silence and unbending blackness; was she going mad? This ring, simply a band of gold was only a token; others had been driven mad by the same in the name of marriage or felicity of another sort. Could she sacrifice another's life, lest her own, just to preserve the lovely unending line, at this point the only true constant in her life. But this ring is for the ages, stretching far beyond the moment. Moist, cool air enveloped the two. Occasional water drips, growing ancient formations, are heard at close range, then... yes, farther away another lake was filling with steady, deliberate drops of water, the lifeblood of this subterranean hiding place. This would be Hades to the ancients, but to the Seekers of Tom it was becoming a heaven, the darkness a balm. Were they dying? No...too close to the legacy's unfolding. Ah, breathe, smell the saturated rock, give in and embrace the dark, sleep maybe, yes, just rest a little, dream. Deep sleep is jarred by a gentle sound, not of water, not even footsteps, but distant music, like earthen chimes...is this her heaven? And where is he?"

10.) Inganteria Moelusteian

He sat silently, listening, straining his ears to hear the slightest ruffle, a sniff, a breath, the faint zip of cloth on flesh, as she moved. He drew the air in deeply and slowly through his nose to avoid any sound. He smelled a woman's scent, the faint waft of this morning's perfume, mixed with the smell of the coffee, that she'd thrown all over him. He raised his hands to his face and gently let his fingertips explore the damage. Already there were fluid filled blisters around his eyes. He didn't know how well he could see, it didn't really matter here anyway. The Tom that they called Frank had written of the olcooedootdso dome, as if that were enough to deceive him, he could decipher that with or without the ring. It was the "code to loose" and he of all Toms knew what it was meant for. It was the antithesis of everything that their order stood for. It would loose the most destructive force on earth, the demons of hope and belief, on all of mankind. Belief lay with the doctor, the one he'd already tried to kill, the Tom that they called Anderson. He'd escaped but the information that Inganteria had found on the computer at his office had led him here, to abolish hope.

Damned hope…hope the most virulent of all curses. And it was this one the one he hunted now that was the key to that hope. He'd seen it in her eyes when he had grabbed her to stab her. She'd never even seen the knife, she'd lashed out, not in anger, not in rage, not even in the paranoia that was engulfing the entire world now, but with hope. The hope that she could escape. The hope that she could survive this to see her husband again, to raise their children. It had burned him to the core of his soul.

She was nearby, the answer was to wait, the first one to move loses.

11.) Ambush

Frank: Tom was laying in the bushes, M16 trained on the caves entrance....the MD 20/20 really tasted good after the fight he had with the gypsies over the secret decoder ring....damn gypsies tried to lie and say the ring was 'lost'. Frank (Tom) put one of the gypsies down....maybe for good. Now, sipping the 20/20, he was about to put another, possibly two down. He hoped he didn't have to, but .... some things just have to be done....

His mind drifted to the past, when he trusted MS CGS and Inganteria. How could he be so stupid.......so blind.....Rain started falling lightly now, it was cold....and fog was starting to set in..............

Eavesdropping

It's not nice to eavesdrop. We all grew up with that admonition. If your parents caught you lurking around in the hall while they were discussing something in whispered tones about the new neighbors, you were pretty sure that you were going to get whopped in the back of the head, told to knock it off, and if it was still light, sent out into the back yard. I tell my kids that.

"Do you want people to think you're creepy, or something?"

"No."

"Then don't eavesdrop, it's creepy."

I don't whop them much any more, it's too much trouble with girls. Besides these kids need all the brain cells they can keep.

So, we're all in agreement here. Eavesdropping is not nice, it's creepy, it's sneaky, and a whole bunch of other bad stuff, unless of course, you're a parent, and then it's essential.

Listening in has always been the parent's main source of information about what's happening. What kind of stuff happened that day at school, who did what to who, who cheated on a test, all the stuff you need to know. For you newer parents, the best time to eavesdrop is in the car. You can hear everything they say. And if you've got the technique down, which is to never butt in or mention anything that you overhear until later, your kids think you're too deaf to hear them. So they keep on talking like you're not even there. Several times I've mentioned something I've overheard in the car later in the evening, and had a kid say, "Where'd you hear about that?"

Charlene had a pat answer, "The mother network." The kids never questioned it. See, I told you we needed to preserve as many brain cells as possible.

Unfortunately, all that's changing with this last bunch of kids we're raising. They don't talk that much in the car anymore. They text. All you can hear is clickety click click click, clickety click. If you're like me you don't have any idea what all the clicks mean or even why they're texting one another when they're sitting right next to each other in the car. My two daughters do that constantly. They'll be sitting right next to each other on a bench type seat in the back of the car and start having a texting argument. As the driver parent you have no idea what they're doing or even that they're fighting until one of them eventually screams.

"Sissy texted me a brat!"

Of course, being the wise benevolent father that I am, I have the perfect solution.

"Put those stupid phones up or I'm going to throw them out of the window."

"If you throw my phone out the window, can I get an I-phone?"

"Of course not, why would I get you an I-phone if I had to throw your phone out of the window?"

"What about the new Blackberry?"

"NO! Now put 'em up!"

"I don't know why I can't have internet service?"

"Because you're ten. What do you need to get on the internet for anyway?"

"To go on Facebook."

"You're not allowed to go on Facebook."

"I could if you got me an I-phone."

"No you can't…"

You get the idea, see, in the past you would have spent all that time socking away valuable bits of parental intelligence, now it's wasted on electronic warfare.

My wife objects to using warfare related terms to describe parenting techniques. I don't know why. The way I look at it they (the children and sometimes I think my wife,) are trying to kill me. That's why they say these things, to try and give me a stroke. I don't know if they're working individually or collectively. That's another reason I have to eavesdrop on them.

But sometimes it's purely for the entertainment of it. I love to listen to my children play. Tonight was a classic. Maddie and Holton were in the next room. I'm not sure what they were playing. Maddie was a lady with a horse farm and the horses. Holton was apparently a general and an alien invader.

Lady voice: "I'm going to town to get some hay for supper. Does anyone want to go with me?"

Horse voice: "Neigh neigh. I do. I do."

General voice: "Battlefield command request permission to launch a rocket strike on this location to destroy the aliens."

Alien voice: "They're requesting an air strike. We have to deploy the disrupters."

Maddie: "What are you doing? We're playing horses."

Holton: "I know, but the horses are stuck in the middle of an interplanetary conflict."

Maddie: "You can't launch rockets if horses are in the way."

General voice: "I'll clarify that. Launch control, launch control we have livestock on the battlefield. I repeat livestock on the battlefield."

Reply: "General, this is the president. I repeat this is the president. Launch your rockets...launch your rockets. We cannot let the safety of the world be endangered by livestock.

Maddie: "Holton that's *not* the way you play horsies. Besides, what kind of idiot president would let them blow up horses? You didn't even tell him they were horses, you said livestock. He probably thought they were pigs."

General voice: "I'll get further clarification. Blue Eagle, Blue Eagle, this is Sly Fox One. The livestock in question are horses, I repeat, not pigs, horses."

Reply: "General you have your orders. It is sure a shame that the horses have to die, but we can build a statue to the brave horses that gave their lives to save the world."

Maddie: "You and your army are a bunch of idiots. I'm going to be with the aliens."

Alien voice: "Save the horses. We eat them for desert on our planet."

Maddie: "What kind of planet eats horses?"

Holton: "You're so stupid. Ours does. They make them into dog food too."

WHAP

Holton: "Owww owww owww. You're not allowed to hit people with the horses, they're hard."
Me: "Maddie you better not be hitting anybody with those horses."
Maddie: "I didn't. The horses were just defending theirselves."

Just another slice of my life.

Connect the Dots

You know you're just a passenger,
that's passing on your way,
Still trying to figure out what you can do,
to blunt the pain today?

She glides gracefully, feeling the wind slide over her wings. The air taking the longer path over the dome of her wing keeping her aloft. She's one with the sky, until she spots what it is she's been looking for. She adjusts the tension in her left wing to correct her course, staying high, staying high until it's almost too late. And then she drops. Talons out, extended, open. Bracing for the shock of contact.

His name was Hugh Hefner. He'd heard the jokes his whole life. He wouldn't hear them much longer.

Wheeling, wheeling almost too high to believe, she could see where the pine forests gave way to a small clearing with a tar paper shack in the middle of it.

Billy let his fingers slide along the sharp metal strings. It was a kid's guitar, a little Yamaha, the neck was too narrow for his big old fingers, but he didn't guess it mattered much any more if he buzzed a note or muffed a chord. His fingers caressed the guitar neck. There'd been a hundred others, all gone now, and he'd never found the key he was looking for, the key out. At least he didn't have to go back to the paper mill again.

He stopped playing for a minute and took a deep drag off of the cigarette between his lips. He held his breath for as long as he could, which wasn't very long, before he let the smoke trickle out of his nose. It had been more fun at eighteen. He inhaled again. Smokin' dope and playing guitar. He'd used to think he could see his future when he got high back then. He sighed as he let the smoke back out of his lungs. It just didn't quite turn out the way he'd seen it back then. He laid the joint down in the ashtray and went back to playing.

He started in on *El Camino Dolo Rosa*, the Mott the Hoople song, it was sad enough and he let the song wind around and around with a few variations each time around, before he let it ease into the rhythm line from *Southbound Again*. He'd liked that first album…

He stopped and took another drag. The ember was almost dead but revived and grew as he drew on it.

"I guess I got eternity to sit here and play, eternity and no time at all both together at the same time," he told it.

He reached for the ashtray. It was time to let this one go out. The heat was burning his lips now. He'd roll another one in a bit. He balanced the ashtray on his leg, but as he turned back to play, the guitar bumped it. It was kind of weird to watch the red tip burn a hole in his pajama pants, the black ring growing, and not feel a damned thing. Couldn't move his leg to shake it off, trying to get his arm out from around the little guitar to smack it off of him. He didn't want holes burned in him if he could feel them or not. He smacked and fell sideways off the bed. The guitar broke as it hit the floor beside him.

She was not so big a bird. Not the bird that would not let it come day. Her powers were small.

Mary was the mother of God, but she didn't feel much like it as she walked down the children's hallway at Central Baptist Church. She was picking her little girl up from the nursery just like her mama had when she still felt like she belonged there. When church was still a holy place. When she was a little girl. Before she changed. Before she'd lost her virginity at fourteen, to Wiley Thomas, in the back of the choir box.

She looked at the sweet-faced Jesus standing in a flock of lambs that reached his hand out to her as she passed the stained glass window. Jesus is supposed to be merciful. If he was so merciful how'd he let her get pregnant by such a worthless shit as Frankie Wright? He hadn't even seen the baby since she was born, and now she was three years old, and he shows up, come in off working the oilrigs in the gulf and saying that he wants custody. Marries that little coonass tramp and now that makes him a daddy. He better hopes Jesus forgives, she thought, cause if it was me, I'd send his ass on the express elevator, straight down to hell. She never saw the Toyota car before it ran through the wall, its gas pedal stuck to the floor. Jesus turned into a million diamonds that all rushed to her at once.

The bird called Death floated up again and flapped just once, before she started to glide, it had been a long day and she was full now. It was time to rest. She'd hunt again tomorrow, but for today, she was done.

A strange little idea that grew and then she flew.

Author's note:

For all of you that didn't, <u>Connect the Dots</u> was a picture of three accidental deaths that presented to an ER in a 24hr period, you explain it how you like, divine providence, random happenstance, whatever. I chose a little bird called death. It seems that for me accidental deaths are so much harder to make sense of than those that we expect, because with those we have been tipped off by the onset and can follow the progression of symptoms. Maybe we just understand that the chronicity of disease has an inevitability about it.

Once I had a patient with an advanced head and neck cancer that was essentially incurable. If the tumor would have killed him, he would have been just as dead. But a piece of tin roofing flying off of a pick-up truck on the highway and cutting off his head just seemed like a different thing, somehow, a more dramatic thing, a worse thing. I don't know why.

This column is another way to look at death, it is the opening of a novel I'm putting out under the pen name Russell Scott called: The Hard Times. It is from a doctor's perspective this time, but maybe a little different viewpoint than you might expect.

Hard

Charlie Lee was pretty sure he wasn't dead yet. He was hurting too badly to be dead, but there was a good chance he was headed in that direction if something didn't change fairly quickly. He was lying face down in the middle of the kitchen floor and he couldn't get up because it felt like somebody had parked a cement truck on top of him. He fought just to breathe, trying with all his strength to lift the truck enough to let his ribs expand, but no matter how hard he tried, it wasn't working.

Not enough oxygen was making its way to his brain. His thoughts began to fade and blur. Then he was on his back. His wife, Millie, was shaking his shoulders and calling his name. For a moment he tried to answer her, but he couldn't do that either. He could see her, in bits and pieces when she was directly over him. In the brief glimpses he got, Charlie could see the panic in her eyes. He wished he could tell her it was going to be all right. That he'd be fine in a minute, if he could only catch his breath.

Instead though, the truck on top of him seemed to be getting heavier every second. Crushing down, down, down, until the weight of the universe was centered in his chest. In that weight was a sudden clarity. His heart wasn't beating. He hadn't paid any attention to it before now. Instead of the steady, lub-dub he never really noticed, he could feel a bag of snakes crawling around inside him.

The pain continued to build, getting worse and worse until he didn't think he could stand it anymore. He rode it like a wave. He didn't have a choice. As a doctor, he'd watched people die for thirty-five years. He knew what it looked like from the outside. Now, he was finding out what it felt like first-hand.

His wife started to blow air into his mouth. The air just blew back out his nose. Then she remembered her CPR and pinched it shut so the air would go into his lungs. The pain got better. Subsiding little by little as she blew into his mouth. Millie dialed the phone between breaths. No answer. She dialed again. What was she doing? Dial 9-1-1, Charlie thought. Somebody's going to answer that. Finally, she spoke to someone and checked his pulse.

"No," she said. "He doesn't"

Then she started to pump on his chest as well, but she was doing it all wrong. The sequences were crazy. There wasn't any rhythm at all. Five pumps-one breath then eight compressions and two breathes. On she went, crying as she did, four-one, seven-two, six-one, eleven-three. It was maddening, but apparently it was working. He was still here wasn't he, he was pretty sure dead people weren't irritated by the irregularity of their wife's chest compressions.

He should have lost some weight. He could feel the fat on his stomach shaking as his wife continued pumping with her erratic rhythms. He was going on a diet when he got through this.

Poor Millie. He could feel her wearing out, pumping slower, having to stop to catch her breath before she could blow into his mouth again. He didn't know if she was going to be able to make it until the ambulance arrived, but somehow she did. He recognized the paramedic's voice. It was Bobby Pierson, from the hospital. He knew what was coming when he heard Bobby yell "clear". Electric shock was the only thing that could stop the chaos that was keeping his heart from beating.

Nothing that you thought you knew could prepare you for what that felt like. The horrible jerking energy threw him out into space. He spun, rigid and awful, away from the world and drifted back just in time to hear Bobby call "clear" again, and it happened all over. This time it was harder and it was taking longer to get back. He never got all the way, because they hit him again before he made it, and he was gone again, somewhere else.

This time he was nowhere, a black speck looking across a blinding plain. Three men moved across the expanse. The man who was closest was alone. He felt familiar somehow, familiar, but beyond recognition, faceless in the light. Two other men moved together, coming from far away. He wasn't sure who they were, or why they came towards him. He was where their paths came together. But he wasn't a person anymore or a place. He'd become part of the light itself.

Then, suddenly, he wasn't. He was back in the world. He felt the bumping as they locked him into place in the back of the ambulance, felt his wife's hand. He could hear her voice coming to him. He could tell that she was talking to someone else and then to him. He couldn't see her. He felt her squeeze his hand. Even though he couldn't really make out what it was that she was saying, he began to feel better as he listened to the rhythm of her voice, and he knew that whatever it was that they were doing now, it was working. He wasn't going to die after all. He felt so much better.

Danger-Geenuse At Work

I was twelve when my father graduated from medical school. How he convinced my mother that it was somehow reasonable to leave his job as a pharmacist, with four children, the youngest still a baby, and attend medical school I'll never know. It's well beyond my powers of persuasion, that I'm sure of. But somehow he did. He was at the University of Kentucky. My mom got a job as a secretary in the Civil Engineering Department. He worked as many weekends as he could as a pharmacist and my mother typed term papers in the evenings and on weekends to try to get by. So we weren't poor, but we weren't far from it.

I have to say that this was a formative period in my life. It helped me to develop many useful skills, which would serve me well as I got older. A key factor in my development was my place as the oldest child. I was supposed to keep an eye on the rest of the kids. Now that taught me how to delegate almost immediately. My sister Sherie was only fifteen months younger than I was, and she liked the idea of playing house. So it was a perfect fit. She took care of the younger two and I was left to do all the things that any self-respecting kid without too much supervision would do.

To say that a few of the ideas I came up with were unhealthy or dangerous might be true, but in general the degree of danger depended on what the idea was, and who you were in relation to where the plan was going. Safety was always foremost in my deliberations. Like the time I convinced my little brother, Jim, to put on his winter coat and run around the back yard while I shot at him with my BB gun. At first blush I will admit that this does appear to be a bad and dangerous thing. But you have to take into account that my parents didn't have the money to send me on a real bear hunt, and I wanted to be prepared in case of an unexpected bear attack later in life. In truth, Jim was really in very little danger, as long as I shot straight and hit him in the coat. He just had to keep his hands in his pockets and not duck or jump. Unfortunately, a low BB and an angry mother put an end to my bear hunting practice, but at least I know that if a bear runs around my yard (without ducking or jumping of course) I am prepared.

But, these sort of stories somehow seem to show up at every family gathering as an example of my unsuitability as a big brother. Things start out fine, but I know that before the night is over my wife and kids will be regaled by my ungrateful siblings with exaggerated tales of my childhood atrocities. In truth, none of them could have been all that bad. After all, nobody was maimed or severely disfigured in any of them, and no, a few puney scars or a little temporary memory loss doesn't count as a permanent injury if you think about it.

Not one of my siblings ever bothers to take the time to consider all of the good I did them intellectually.

I am quite sure that if somebody walked up to my brother today and asked him to don a bulletproof vest and run around their yard so they could try to shoot him, that not only would he decline the offer, but that there is a very good chance that he'd probably call them a bunch of pretty rude names to boot. All because of that valuable lesson learned so long ago as a child. Yet does he thank me for the insight he gained from that lesson? Never.

Lest you believe my siblings and think that they were the sole objects of what they derisively call my "crazy schemes" (I prefer to think of them as manifestations of my early genius and adventurous spirit) I can cite numerous instances of crazy schemes in which no other family members were injured or even involved, for that matter.

Take for example, the time a bunch of us boys got a wire cage from the concrete pipe factory, and then used our belts to lash one of our friends, Davey, into place so he could travel safely. Then we rolled him down the railroad tracks on a long downgrade.

Davey was the daredevil of our little neighborhood gang, so it was natural that Daredevil was his favorite comic book character. Now Daredevil was a blind guy that fought crime by swinging around the city with a whip and using his karate skills and his whip to whip bad guy's butts, as it were. Davey's mother still kind of blamed the rest of us, and me in particular, for that concussion he got when he tried to show us how he could swing from branch to branch is the big oak tree in my back yard with the new bullwhip he got on a trip to the Smokey Mountains.

Davey, never content at action alone, had decided that if he was going to act like a super-hero he needed to dress the part as well. So, he went home and put on one of those Speedo type bathing suits we all had as kids, except they came from J. C. Penny. His was blue and from last summer, so it was way too tight. He swiped a red stretch top of his big sister's with ruffles on the collar and put that on too. He tied one of his mom's white bath towels around his neck, and put on a pair of black cowboy boots, then came clomping back across the yards. I had to admit that he sure looked like a super-hero dressed like that, popping that whip in the air…CRACK.

He climbed up into the tree and got out on one of the main branches, put his hand on his hip, and announced, "I am Daredevil. The boy without fear."

"Alright, boy without fear, that's wearing his sister's shirt, let's see ya swing on that whip like you said you could." I said, mad that Connie the really cute little girl that lived between us, had told my sister how great Davey looked dressed up like that.

He bowed to the girls and they tittered. "Damned showoff." I mumbled.

He started off like gangbusters. He snapped that whip around a fat branch. Tugged on it. It was secure as could be. Then he swung straight out parallel to the ground with those shiny black boots pointing at the sky and his "cape" trailing behind him. He was looking like a real super-hero. Right up until the whip broke and he fell twelve feet and landed flat on the back of his head. He didn't move for a real long time so I had to run down the street and get his mom.

One of the things I remember most about Mrs. Mullins, was how fast she was, for an older woman. She'd go tearing off across the neighbor's yards, muttering "not again," under her breath and not even panting. I had to run about as fast as I could just to keep up.

By the time we got there Davey was starting to mumble something, so he obviously wasn't dead, which made me take a sigh of relief. I looked at his mom and she had a really strange look on her face, kind of a mix of scared, and mad, and about to laugh all at the same time.

"Do you want to try and explain to me why my son is dressed up like this?" She demanded.

Now I've been a kid <u>and</u> a parent and there's one thing I can tell you;

there is just no use in asking questions like this. If you can't make sense of it on the face of things, you can be pretty sure you're not going to get a straight answer from a kid, particularly one that might possibly incriminate himself in some way.

"He said he was Daredevil, the boy without underwear." I answered, trying to get even for the girls thinking he looked so cute.

Then all those girls started chiming in, saying that wasn't it at all…they jabbered all the way back to his house, and the whole time while his mom loaded him up in the car for another quick trip to the Emergency Room.

I never really got specifically blamed. And Davey got to stay off school for a whole week. So I guess things turned out the best that they could have. Except that Davey wasn't allowed to come outside to play in the afternoons for a while, and his mom threw the bullwhip and his bathing suit away, but it could have been a lot worse. And I for one wasn't that sad to see that bathing suit go, no matter what the girls said.

It was Davey's own choice to ride that cage we rolled down the train tracks. I just bet him he was too chicken to do it, but I was sure wrong. He climbed right in and we all took off our belts so we could safety belt him in place. Watching that cage spin down the tracks, I was in awe of how far he'd got without throwing up. We were all whooping and hollering and pounding each other on the back and saying how brave Davey was, when a low sorrowful wail drifted up to us from across the river. As we watched him going along straight as an arrow down the tracks every one of us knew that what we were hearing was the whistle of an oncoming train. At first we were stupefied, the train wasn't supposed to go through there for another twenty minutes.

Then we started running. We ran as fast as we could but we were still losing ground, as the rolling cage hit the steep part of the downgrade and accelerated down the hill away from us. I guess Davey heard the whistle too. I'm surprised he could hear anything personally. But he did and he started thrashing around like crazy trying to get his hands and feet loose from those belts we'd tied him in with. He wasn't having much luck. We'd belted him in good and tight so he didn't have to worry about getting hurt again and getting his mom mad at all of us all over again. The last thing we wanted was him smashing his fingers or something.

Anyway, all that fighting to get loose from the belts got the cage off balance. It came off one rail then we all watched as it flipped sideways down the embankment and flew thirty or forty feet before it hit the ground. He was still a good way before he reached the trestle. But we kept on running just in case he'd gone into the river or the creek that fed into it.

It was slow going when the train got there, because we had to get off to the side to let it pass. Davey had been real lucky though. He was nice and safe in that blackberry patch that was just above the creek bank. He did look like he'd come out on the losing end of a fight with a dozen bobcats. Nothing a little Mercurochrome couldn't fix, and no trip to the Emergency Room this time.

Again, a valuable lesson was learned that would serve Davey well the rest of his life and he was barely injured learning it.

I, myself, was not immune to the adverse effects of an active intellect. One of the many instances of this that comes to mind also involved Davey. His family was a little better off than we were, and Davey was the baby of six kids, so he got everything cool. At this particular point in time one of the coolest things in existence was a StingRay bicycle with front extension forks, so you could ride leaning back. I had a good bike, it was a Schwinn Loadmaster or something with twenty-eight inch wheels, and weighing in at about a hundred pounds. If you fell over it seemed like it took about a week to hit the ground. It was great to use on my magazine delivery route, but it wasn't cool.

The fact that Connie would sit on the curb in front of her house and make "ooohing" and "aaahhing" sounds while Davey popped wheelie after wheelie, was just like rubbing salt in a wound. I tried popping a couple of wheelies on the Loadmaster. Throwing the whole of my seventy five pounds into jerking the handle bars up, resulted in little if any discernable effect on the bikes front wheels. The welded steel front package rack may have had something to do with that, I don't know. But the decision was made. I had to come up with a cooler bike, even if I had to build it myself.

I knew a place down by the creek where there was a kid's bike frame. So I pulled that out. After I washed it off as good as I could, it wasn't as rusty as I first thought. A couple of coats of flat black paint from my dad's tool shed did the trick perfectly. I traded a pocket knife for a banana seat and used my magazine money to buy a set of "ape-hanger" handle bars, but it took every penny I had. There was no money left for the extension forks.

I had to have the extension forks, that's what the girls thought was so cool.

I had made my pseudo-StingRay from junk, I had a skateboard made from a skate and a board, there had to be a way for me to get some extension forks. I was just going to have to think of a way to do it myself. I made a trip a few houses down and "liberated" a pole from Mrs. Watson's clothesline. Then used a hacksaw to cut it in half, and a hammer to flatten the ends. I drilled holes in the flattened ends so the axel bolts fit through, tightened them down, then flipped the bike over and hammered the free ends of the poles onto the forks of the bike. A little more black spray paint and…Viola, the coolest bike around.

I can't begin to tell you how smart I felt riding around on my own bike for the next three or four days, popping wheelies and acting too cool to notice Connie sitting there with my sister. Then it all fell apart…literally.

The days of riding around had loosened the hold the hammered on aluminum poles had on the front forks of the bike. I popped one wheelie too many and the whole contraption fell off. I kept pumping to keep the bike from throwing me face first into the asphalt. There was no way to let the bike down and the more I pumped the faster I was going. Consequently, the more it was going to hurt when I did hit the asphalt.

Luckily a kindly bread truck was crossing the intersection as I ran the red light and I smashed into the side of it breaking my arm. The bike wasn't so lucky. It went under the back wheels and looked kind of like a metal pretzel after that.

What valuable insight did I gain from this? I guess that the best way to say it is that just because you <u>can</u> do something, it doesn't always mean that you should. That lesson stuck with me for quite a while…well, until that unfortunate incident with the electric drill and the gas grill that just happened to blow up right after I drilled those holes in it. My mustache and eyebrows only took a month or so to grow back. I'll keep you posted on any other valuable lessons I can come up with.

Author's Note: It's a good story so I included it, but it was a whole lot less amusing for me after my little brother Jim died this summer. I wish I'd have been a better brother to him as a child. But there's no changing the past, so I'm sure he's going to whip up some surprise to get me back if I ever make it to heaven. He deserves to. I've earned whatever it is I get.

A Free Man

I'm back. Yep, I met with the Editor and they've decided to keep me on. So I'll be writing this thing for another year. I guess that's good, or bad maybe, depending on if you like the stuff I write, or not.

This year will be a little different though, for the first time since I started stringing together words for the JOURNAL I'm unencumbered. Well, I'm still encumbered by nutty thoughts that ping around in my brain, but what I mean to say is I'm not tied to the association by any official strings. I've finished my term on the board of trustees and am no longer on the AMA delegation.

It's just me, so if I say stuff you don't like, you're welcome to hold it against me but you shouldn't expect I'll lose a lot of sleep at night just because you think I'm an idiot. I'm used to that. I have a whole family that thinks I'm an idiot from time to time.

The unencumbered stuff is only partly an accident, I guess. Most of it was my own doing. I did run to be re-elected to our rapidly diminishing AMA delegation…I lost, but I got to give one of the most fun to give campaign speeches I could ever imagine giving.

It was one of those things that comes to you when you're driving a pretty long way, like Meridian to Tupelo, and you have time to let things roll around inside your head, getting bigger and bigger as you drive. Usually, after you get to wherever it is that you're going, common sense takes over and you write a real speech, but I didn't get that chance. See I'd had to run back home in the middle of the meeting to treat an emergency patient, an old friend, who'd developed a spinal cord compression in the mid-thorasic spine. Not wanting them to be paralyzed from the waist down for what life they had left, there wasn't a lot of choice. Anyway I got back to Tupelo, got out of the car and gave the speech, about that fast. Here it is, as best as

I remember:

Our inaugural theme for this year is "A Night at the Races", so in keeping with that theme, I'm going to talk about this election in racing terms. See, as far as medical politics goes, the AMA meeting is the Kentucky Derby. It's our chance to shine in the national spotlight, and up to now we have. You, the Mississippi State Medical Association, are the riders, and we, the AMA delegation have been the horse that runs the race. Well, next year you've decided that it will be best for Mississippi to enter the Kentucky Derby riding on a two-legged pig.

By quitting the AMA you've left your delegation with only one delegate and one alternate delegate. That makes our delegation the same size as the delegations from Puerto Rico, and the gay and transgender physician section.

So what this election is all about is deciding what two legs you think you need on that pig. Do you want a couple of hams? We surely have our share of hams on the delegation. We can harness the power of those hams and go plowing along through the dirt trying to get around the track. Maybe we need a couple of strong shoulders, we have plenty of those on the delegation too, a little more dignified perhaps. They can pull us along. Or maybe you all want one ham and one shoulder. We can try to find a way to balance ourselves and not fall over in the dirt.

None of these, I submit, is a good alternative. It is a shame is what it is. You want to tell me that the AMA doesn't represent you, that the delegation isn't important to you? Well the work of this delegation is directly responsible for you getting checks for 8.1% of your entire gross federally derived income last year. By fighting to require CMS to abide by the congressionally mandated geographic price correction we prevailed. That meant something to you. You put that money in your pocket. Nobody called to say, "I'm not taking this damned money, the AMA got it, and I don't approve of the AMA." Destroying this delegation, just to make a political point, when you're benefitting from the work that it does is shortsighted and stupid.

My friends have told me that this is a suicide speech. If it is...then so be it. Somebody has to tell you the truth. If we get 1001 members of this association, one fourth of our membership, to re-join the AMA, at least we'd have two delegates and two alternates. While we still probably won't win the Kentucky Derby on a four-legged pig, I'm betting we'll eat a lot less dirt.

It was a great time. I got to pound on the lectern and point at people and tell the truth. Who could possibly ask for more?

The election turned out fine. We decided on two strong shoulders, I couldn't have asked for a better outcome…unless, of course, those of you out there reading this listen to what it is I've said, and do what it's going to take to get us a couple more legs to run on.

See ya next time,
One of the hams

Portrait of a Two-Lane Road

My son, Dylan and I have always loved to travel around by a method we refer to as "heading in the general direction." This is no dead reckoning, it does not involve Mapquest directions or GPS coordinates. It does not involve interstates, unless we need to use them for a while, or they're the most direct route to get us to somewhere else we want to meander around. I started it with him so he could derive a confidence in his ability to get from one place to another, one way or another. That doesn't mean you won't hit a dead end or a dirt road once in a while, but you learn to turn around, backtrack a little and keep on moving toward your destination. We went to lots of sporting events and camps this way before he could drive, I'd let him pick which roads we turned on and then tell him why or why not it might be a good idea. Things like, don't aim straight at a big body of water, or only take roads you can see are paved above or below you on a mountain. When he could drive we'd headed over to east Texas to pick up a dog that way. Once we even flew up to Fayetteville, Arkansas to pick up a 1966 Mustang with no spare car, no trailer, and no real plan except to drive home.

Even before Dylan was old enough to join in, that was how I drove whenever time permitted. I even managed to cross the United States that way, both back and forth, and up and down one time. It was when I completed my residency in Norfolk, Virginia and was ordered to report to my next duty station in San Diego. I came out of residency with about a hundred and forty days of leave on the books. The most you were allowed to carry on reporting for duty was ninety. As soon as I reported in, the Navy would rob me of the additional fifty days, and I didn't see any reason to just give them up, so I got sixty days leave and travel time authorized and set off across the country. Now I don't care how slowly you drive, it doesn't take sixty days to get across the continental United States. Since my orders didn't allow me to leave them, I figured I'd have to zigzag some along the way, but that's another story for another time.

Anyway, back to what I originally intended to talk about. It all started because it was the first of June and I was up in Oxford. I'd just finished attending this year's annual session of the Mississippi State Medical Association and had a three hour drive south back home to Meridian. It was a beautiful Sunday morning and there was nobody at home waiting for me. Between rodeos, golf, and tennis camp, everybody was gone somewhere. So, I just needed to get home sometime, not at any particular time, and it was just too damned pretty to drive straight.

I decided to head in the general direction of home, but if I was going to do much two-lane driving on the way, I knew I needed to do it above Starkville, unless I wanted to end up in Philadelphia. Now I don't have anything against Philadelphia, but I've been there a lot and I've traveled most of the roads from Philadelphia to either my home in Meridian or to our farm in Newton enough that I don't really consider it too much fun anymore. There just aren't all that many surprises left. I pretty much know the roads, the houses, and even most of the horses along the way.

My plan was to head south on County 9 out of Oxford toward Bruce. That's how I planned to start anyway, somewhere I'd turn east to Houlka, and angle south again toward Houston and end up on Highway 45 near West Point.

That was the plan when I turned the engine over but now it's just me and the car. As we come up over a little hill eight or nine miles down the road, I see a left that looks attractive so I turn. The little road is kind of like a Dalmatian, all spotted. It isn't rough or bad at all, the county had done a good job with it, but it's just about as much hot-patch as there is original asphalt. I look off to the right as I roll along a good straight stretch and see an impossibly bright sap green field. A baby blue valve head is sticking out of the ground right in the middle of the field. As I move across it the sun glints off of the shiny new looking silver pipe that the valve is sitting on top of. It's so bizarre, everything anywhere around the field, the house, the barn, even the fence is worn out and busted down, and there's that blue valve and shiny pipe sticking up, with the cattle grazing all around it. They don't even notice it. I guess they think "maybe it grew there," if they think at all.

That's one of my problems. I can't stop thinking. Sometimes I wish that I was one of those cows, and that nothing would strike me as strange or worry me. That's one of the reasons I like the two-lane. I don't think about any of the things that worry me, I don't think about what I should do next. Everywhere I go on the two-lane I only think one thing, over and over. I always think, "I should paint that," but then, I roll along around the next bend and see something else that grabs my imagination, and then I forget all about what it was I wanted to paint a minute ago, and I think, "I should paint that."

It happens again this time. As soon as I get past the field with the blue valve on the silver pipe with all peaceful cows eating, I see a black dog lying next to a Lincoln with a dark purple top and lavender body underneath a huge live oak. It's very dramatic in its contrast, but in all honesty, I don't guess that I'll ever have a car painted like that for myself. But it's gone now. I see a smattering of red up ahead in a stand of new green saplings and wonder what kind of plant might it be that's growing in there. As I come on around, I can see that it's not a plant at all, that the red is rust, on an old tin roof. It's on a faded white house that people haven't lived in for some time. The floorboards are caved in and smaller saplings sprout up through the gaps in the floor to grow on the porch. People'd sat on that porch, in years past. I don't know if they were white people or black people, but I could imagine them there, sitting on the porch on a day like today, the temperature up around ninety, sipping tea and wishing for a cool breeze to blow on by. I blow by and wave to the king snakes and termites that live there now.

I see a big hawk on a power line,. He's being harried by a catbird or a mockingbird. I can't tell from this distance, but the hawk's had enough. He launches and flaps slowly, the smaller bird following him plucking at his feathers. I'm so engrossed in watching this play out that I almost hit a big snapping turtle that somebody else already has. He looks like an army helmet on the head of a soldier that's been shot, the exploded carapace with bright red shooting out of it in every direction.

Up we come, over another hill, and there it is. The next road's there on the right. I don't know what road it is or where it goes; I just know it's the next one. I'm going too fast, so I brake hard. I haven't seen another car going in either direction for the last ten minutes, and there's a little gravel on the road, so I hang out the tail and let the car slide sideways for a bit before the big tires bite and we go shooting right. I've almost overshot the turn, so I have to come back a bit, cutting across some grass and the wrong lane to do it, but we're okay.

In a big brown field, there's a small white church. It's not much bigger than a utility shed, but the doors are open and spilling out of the darkened interior is a profusion of black faces surrounded by every color of the rainbow, casserole dishes and bibles in their hands, the children sprinting in front of the grown-ups across the dirt parking lot. And then they're gone, as I go flashing by.

I see a white man in a sweat ringed yellow shirt; it hangs on him wet and stifling, even from the car. White bony legs poke up out of black rubber boots that end just below the knobs of his knees. He's swinging an orange weed-eater; a Husquavarna, or a Stihl I'd guess, but even as he works he takes the time to raise his hand and wave to me as I go rushing by. I wave back and smile. *U. S. Blues* is playing on the radio, and I think that this is what Uncle Sam looks like to me, or maybe it's God. I don't know. Just an old man weed-eating in those black boots on the weekend.

My bladder is starting to let me know it's still there and not as happy as it might be, if I wouldn't have had that fourth cup of coffee before I left. A good left is coming up, it's a bigger road and should have a gas station on it somewhere, so I take it. I start to pass cars hauling boats going in the other direction. There must be a lake or something around here.

I pull into a little store/bait shop with a gas pump out front and make my way to the rest room. Coming out, I grab a Diet Coke and walk up to the counter. Two girls sit behind it, the younger of them is about thirteen, she has on cut off jeans and a T-shirt. She's at that awkward stage. She's started to put on a little weight, but it doesn't know where to go yet and her clothes are too tight in this heat. She'll be prettier in a few years, you can tell by the older girl who looks to be her sister. They're watching a little TV on a card table and sitting on plastic chairs. The older girl gets up as I sit that Coke down and start fishing in my pockets for money. She looks at me. I'm still wearing what I had on at the meeting and my nametag with its ribbons is still on my shirt.

"You're kind of dressed up to be going to the lake," she says.

"I'm just trying to go home." I reply smiling.

"You lost?" The younger girl asks.

"I'm not really lost, but I don't know where I am, if that's what you mean." I answered.

"You're nowhere mister, that's where you are. You're right in the middle of nowhere." The older girl said with a sad downward turn of the corner of her mouth.

I smile at her again and think as I leave, "A time will come, a time <u>will</u> come when you wish with all your heart to be back in this nowhere again."

Back on the road I see more things; the pure, pure, white of three newborn Charolais calves laying on a green hillside; the red bed-slat ribs of a sorrel horse, starving to death in the middle of all this grass because his teeth need to be floated; and I see more things. More than I can tell you. As I close in on Highway 45 and take a right onto the four-lane I whisper.

"I love you nowhere." And I know. When I'm gone from here, and I'm not with you any more, that that's where I'll be. Nowhere.

Doc A's Top Ten List on Nutrition

Well the New Year's here and everybody's finished rushing around for the holidays, the left-overs are finally all eaten up and it time to get serious about the same thing we get serious about every New Year, losing some of that extra weight. If you're wondering what makes me a weight loss expert, I guess I've got two good qualifications. First I'm a doctor, and doctors are supposed to know about losing weight, second, I've lost about six hundred pounds over the years. Now it always seems to find its way back somehow, but I lost it. I am happy because I'm starting this year about four pounds lighter than I did last year, and any year you went down you didn't go up, so that's good.

Well, out of the goodness of my heart I decided that I'd give y'all the benefit of my vast, and growing, knowledge on the subject of nutrition, just to help you along. So pretend you're watching The Late Show with David Letterman and let's get to the top ten.

#10. For all of you moms out there - Cheetos are not a vegetable. A sandwich and Cheetos is not really what you should consider a balanced meal. Kids love them and so do I but a vegetable they are not.

9. Kids – Although it may look like it, broccoli is not really poisonous. I'm sure your mother isn't really trying to kill you by making you eat it. P.S. – don't stick it up your nose so you don't have to eat it, I spent a long evening in an Emergency Room one night trying to get snot covered broccoli out of a three-year – old,

and it wasn't that much fun for either one of us.

8. Okay Dads it's your turn – A diet that's mostly bacon is too high in fat and sodium. Now bacon is good with eggs, on some potatoes, in a salad, on a burger and so on, but try to see if you can cut it back as much as possible, and I know it sounds ridiculous but eating thirty or forty strips of bacon a day isn't a diet. I don't care what Dr. Atkins says.

#7. This one is a pretty universal rule – If you eat enough calories to support a six hundred pound hog for long enough you're gonna start to look like one after a while.

#6. There are a couple of things about eating healthy you may need to think about – for one, switching to a lot of fresh vegetables all at once can lead to the occasional poisonous gas attack, so I wouldn't plan a three hour trip on a church bus until you see how your bowels are holding out.

#5. Another thing, you couples need to be aware that weight loss may do more for your sex life than Viagra can. So you may want to wear a big bathrobe around after you take a shower if you haven't put the kids to bed yet.

#4. There is such a thing as too much salt, and if you eat too much salt you get high blood pressure. And even though your eyes may not actually shoot out of your head and roll around on the floor like you see in cartoons, it still isn't good for you.

#3. Here in Mississippi we eat too much. If folks in Mississippi only ate what they needed, the extra food left over could end hunger in most average size African countries.

#2. People in China mostly aren't too fat, but a Chinese Buffet isn't a diet either. What the average Mississippian eats at a Chinese Buffet could feed a family in China for more than a week.

And the #1 nutrition fact is if you look at yourself in pictures and you look too fat you probably are. I was looking at the Christmas cards my wife sent out, and even though I'm a lot thinner in two-dimensions, I'm still too fat. I guess I better go back through the other nine a few more times myself.

Canine Behavior

I will admit that I'm not an expert on dogs. I've always had at least one dog around if I was here in the United States. I've even trained a few bird dogs, but I don't sit around much and think about what dogs think about. I got the chance to learn a lot about behavior, both human and canine, that I never knew before during a conversation that I had with an eight-year-old recently at a family get-together.

Because the nature of this conversation is potentially embarrassing, the identity of the specific eight-year-old is a secret. A secret, that to avoid being in "deep trouble, with somebody that's gonna be nine soon" I must carry with me to my grave. In fact, to avoid any possibility of the specific eight-year-old being identified I should probably assume the posture of our military when discussing nuclear weapons, by saying that, "I can neither confirm nor deny the presence of an eight-year-old, of any type or description, as having been a part of this conversation."

The promise of anonymity that I made when I asked if I could write about our conversation was secured by that most sacred of vows, a "pinky swear." And everybody knows what happens to somebody that breaks a "pinky promise."

Actually, I didn't, but I wanted to convey the fact that I had a grasp of the serious nature of our agreement, so I shook my head solemnly and affirmed that I would never want to risk that. I could only assume that it must be something horrible in the mind of an eight-year-old child, like having to go to school in your underwear or having to kiss the teacher. (For those of you, who are married to a teacher, remember, I'm qualifying this by saying "in the mind of an eight-year-old child," as I don't wish to offend anyone. I'm sure that kissing your wife would be far from horrible and probably be quite wonderful, not that I'm saying I want to kiss your wife,

The Uncommon Thread

but you get my point).

As it turned out I was wrong, and the consequences were of a far graver nature. I surveyed my children on the subject, and they looked at me as if I had asked them what the purpose of a television set was. The answer was universal.

"Nobody will ever trust you again...duh."

Which to me is significantly worse that going to school in your underwear, and certainly worse than kissing a teacher.

This extremely delicate conversation began with a simple statement: "If I was a dog, I'd tell all the other dogs to sniff my butt." The child said without preamble, lying on the floor on their back and looking up at the ceiling fan.

"You better hush up, and stop being rude. You're going to get in trouble." I responded from the couch.

"No. I was thinking about this, and I'm serious."

"Okay then." I said, still suspicious. "What makes you say that?"

"See there are three kinds of dogs..."

"There are lots of kinds of dogs." I corrected.

"I'm not talking about collies, and poodles, or any of that stuff. I'm talking about how they act."

"Different dogs act different ways." I offered.

"I mean when dogs meet each other they act one of three ways."

"Okay..." I replied, expectantly.

"The first kind of dog runs up and barks and growls and acts all mean. It's like he's saying, "I'm the boss, you better do what I say or I'm going to bite you all up."

"So you don't want to be the boss dog?" I asked, truly curious at this point.

"Naaah, the other dogs don't really like him. It's like they're stuck with him, and they just try to get away from him as soon as they can."

"But he's the alpha male, that's what they call him. He's the dog that all the other dogs have to listen to." I instructed.

"They don't listen to him. They just run off and go somewhere else. They go and be with dogs they like."

"But the alpha males are the toughest dogs in the pack. They're the bravest..." I started.

"They aren't really. They're afraid some other dog is tougher, so they don't want to take a chance. They stand in their own yard and act tough, and growl."

"Okay, so what are the other kinds of dogs?" I asked.

"The second kind of dog is the kind I'd hate to be. He's the scared little dog. He just falls over on his back, with his belly up in the air. He's saying, 'Don't eat me. You can if you want, but I wish you wouldn't.' Sometimes they even pee on themselves."

"Well nobody wants to be that kind of a dog." I reinforced. "So what's the last kind?"

"The last kind of dog is the kind of dog I'd be. He just walks up. It's like he is just sticking out his paw to shake hands with the other dogs. He just lets the other dogs sniff at him. He's saying, 'What's up. Guess what I had for dinner last night.' He's the dog all the other dogs like."

"So he's just laid back."

"No, he's really the brave one. He's not afraid of the other dogs. He just lets them come right up to him. If they act bad or bite at him or something then he might get mad, but most of the time he just acts nice and friendly. So if I was a dog, I'd just tell all the other dogs, 'You can sniff my butt.'"

I took a sip of my coffee and thought about it for a moment.

"It's just the butt smelling that..." I started.

"That's not the right way to say it. Humans might have to get that close to smell. A dog can smell you from across the room. That's like waving to someone. It's not just smelling, dogs sniff. "

For some reason, I found that even more disquieting. "If I were a dog, I think I'd stick to smelling them from across the room. It would be a whole lot more sanitary."

"Dogs don't care about stuff being sanitary. They drink out of the toilet. Their favorite things to do are to roll in cow poop, or eat something dead that they found along side the road. You gotta think like a dog, to see what kind of dog you'd be."

I guessed that I'd never know what kind of dog I'd be, because if I was a dog I wouldn't be capable of rational thought or to make a decision based on reason.

"See you're a people doctor…"

I nodded.

"People get to tell you what's bothering them, right?"

"Most of the time." I replied.

"Well, see, dogs can't talk."

"At least, not any dogs I know." I answered.

"So if I'm gonna be a veterinarian, I've got to know how dogs think, otherwise, how am I gonna know what's wrong with them."

"Good point."

The conversation taught me a couple of things. First, never underestimate an eight-year-old. They see things that we adults are too busy for. Second, canine behavior is not too much different than human behavior, a little more disgusting, maybe, but not that different.

How many of us hasn't seen someone so obsequious that you didn't automatically think of a submissive dog laying on it's back, hoping that the big dog doesn't bite it to pieces? Anybody that has watched a televised football game, with all of the pre-game posturing, not much different from barking and growling, has seen the other side of that coin. Most of us aren't all that comfortable with either of these kinds of behaviors. We do our best to get away from people who act like that, so we can go and hang out with folks we like. I guess my young friend hit the nail on the head. The bravest thing any of us can do is to be open to each other, to get close to each other, to take a chance on each other. The mechanisms of social interaction differ, but the principles are the same. So if you want to know what kind of dog I am, I have to say, I'm the kind of dog that still thinks the whole butt-sniffing thing is disgusting, but I will shake your paw.

Tools of the Trade

Part One

There is something almost cyclical in nature when it comes to using an especially historic tool. It means even more if the instrument is something that has at some time belonged to and been used by one of the giants on who's shoulders you yourself stand. It's as close as a man can come to being able to reach across the bounds of time and seize the past in his own hands.

I was reminded of this as I read an account by Professional Hunter Harry Selby about hunting an elephant with the little .275 Rigby that W.D.M. "Karamojo" Bell had used to harvest so many bulls in the early days of the ivory boom in Africa. Selby had been given the rifle as a gift by the famous author Robert Ruark, complete with an inscribed plaque commemorating the event. It's an interesting and nostalgic tale that ends with the little rifle being sold off through Holland and Holland in London by Selby's son, while Selby was still alive. I couldn't comprehend it really. How could you sell something like that?

It was like selling your grandfather's false teeth. Even if you didn't plan on using them yourself, there's something fundamentally wrong about the idea of them being put to use by someone other than your grandfather. The more I thought about it, the more I found myself enraged at the lack of appreciation and understanding that selling such a treasured artifact entailed. I was determined that something had to be done to right such an egregious wrong. Someone had to take up the torch of tradition, and be history's champion. I knew right then and there that that someone was me. This would be my quest, and I set onto it like a Templar after the grail.

Finding the owner of the rifle wasn't as hard as I'd imagined. I tracked him watching carefully for his footprints along that electronic trail we call the Internet. A broken twig caught my attention, the owner had taken the rifle to Botswana on safari in 2009, and much had been made of the event in the shooting press. Seeing it in pictures I could tell how special the little gun was, but why had somebody whittled a hole in the middle of the stock. I read on gathering clues. The hole was to shove a stick in so you could carry it on your shoulder? What idiot would do that? They never heard of a rifle sling in Karamojo? Nobody had a rope?

I switched from tracking the rifle to stalking the owner. I sent him an e-mail. I was cautious, I didn't want to tip my hand and let him know how much I wanted the gun. It read:

> "I saw your gun on the Internet. You probably should go ahead and get rid or it. After shooting that many elephants the barrel is probably pretty shot out. I bet it won't hold a two-inch group from a rest anymore. The hole in the stock is kind of ugly too. If you decide you want to get rid of it, give me a call."

He didn't call. So I changed strategies.

The old fellow that owned the gun now was kind of skittish acting for being such a big time hunter. He looked kind of panicked when I showed up unannounced and knocked on his door at five a.m. one morning to ask if he'd gotten my e-mails.

I didn't get very much time to talk though. The police station must have been less than two blocks away. The squad car was there before he even came back to the door with the gun.

With a restraining order that kept me from ever returning to Manhasset Township, it was pretty clear that there wasn't going to be hardly any way for me to return the gun to Africa to set it free in it's natural environment.

Most people would have become discouraged at this point and told the cosmic forces of the universe to go to hell, but not me, I knew if I just applied a little creative thinking that there had to be some other way to set things right. I'd just have to do something else, something equally important. Something just as symbolic as getting Bell's gun back to the wild, away from the domestic captivity of a gun safe in New England.

Maybe I could return some other famously historic stupid ugly gun? Again I ran into the stumbling block of financial restraint. All of the famous guns I found cost too much money. I'm all for returning balance to the universe, but let's be reasonable…I have a wife, and spending the price of a new Mercedes on a gun wasn't going to go over all that well. There had to be something else. There was direction being provided here, a message in the failures. Finally, after several weeks of obsessive deliberations, finally I got it. I wasn't a professional hunter. I didn't need a famous gun. I am a writer and a physician. I needed a tool that reflected my own profession's traditions. My grail was defined by who I was, not a scratched and beat up old gun with a hole in it.

My first try involved Hemmingway's whiskey, which I must say was quite enjoyable at first. But the extensive training required to meet Papa's standard of consumption began to have an adverse effect on my ability to hit much of anything at all with a weapon of any type (not to mention the fact that I don't have a lighthouse next to my house to guide my way back from the bar each night). After I almost shot a toe off with a bow and arrow one afternoon after one Daiquiri too many, the die was cast. This was not the right quest either. The crushing headaches I was getting every morning had to be another sign that it was time to move on. Going to rehab for the next two or three months was probably not what was needed to restore balance to the universe anyway.

I'll spare you the details of Mark Twain's pencil, if any one finds it (it's the one with the bite marks that I left in that diner in Joplin), I'd like to have it back, and Roosevelt's glasses (I couldn't see a damned thing I was shooting at). It finally came down to a cockroach in a bottle of formaldehyde, with a paper label that read F. Kafka or Marty Steiner's Underwood. Now Marty wasn't as famous as some of these other folks, but he had known my aunt, and wrote wonderful articles in the Cincinnati Enquirer newspaper a few years ago about going to Africa during the war.

I weighed my options carefully, and couldn't come up with any possible way to use a pickled roach to hunt at all, even if it was named Gregor, and Underwood had made some wonderful rifles for our troops to use in the war, so it was me and the Underwood, off to Africa in pursuit of an elephant.

Part Two

I sat in the bar at the Kalahari Sands Hotel. We were having a couple of sundowners, even though it was only two-o-clock in the afternoon. I didn't think it would hurt anything. It was still the middle of the night back home anyway. I was explaining to John, the professional hunter I'd gotten to agree to guide me on my unusual quest, that it was because of my earnest desire to avoid adversely impacting the elephantine genetic make-up of the Caprivi that I thought we should try to find the oldest and most debilitated animal possible. One that was way, way out of the gene pool, probably best if we even found one that clearly had no possible chance of ever reproducing again.

I blathered on, feeling badly about the whole thing. For all my high flung rhetoric I knew it wasn't a loss of pachyderm genes that was worrying me. It was a lack of confidence. I wasn't sure of myself and I wasn't sure of my weapon. The old Brits called it a case of the nerves.

I let a bit of quiet slide into the conversation and looked glumly at the ice melting in the dregs of gin in the bottom of my glass. Big old balls of elephant dung…there wasn't anything wrong with wanting to take a few precautions, was there? Even Bell had probably knocked off a few gimp elephants before he started blasting the big ones with that ugly little peashooter he made so famous.

The old hunter looked across his glass and held his feelings to himself. I did detect a trace of a frown though when I asked if he knew of any blind or three-legged animals in the area we were going to be hunting in.

We cut tracks on day two; a profusion of deep ovals crossed the dust of the road and trailed into a thick stand of scrub. I leaned on the fender and watched as the two trackers we had with us tried to decipher the meaning in the tracks. When they pushed each other's shoulders and laughed John, who clearly knew their ways well, only nodded with a wry smile. They never spoke.

"See that set?" He asked and pointed out a deep furrow. "Paralyzed leg."

I knew we were onto the right prey. But it was no easy quest. We tracked for the next two hours through the thick thorn brush. The dust coated my mouth. I could use a swig of the gin we'd had at the hotel now.

The elephants track was wide enough to allow us to pass shoulder to shoulder without difficulty, but even at that I left the Underwood cased and in the possession of one of the trackers as we walked. There was no discussion of shoving a stick into it.

Coming around a turn I found John and the two trackers squatted down, eyes hard on an opening in front of us. I eased forward, my eyes straining to see through the brush. With each step I could feel my heart beating ever harder in my throat.

I couldn't swallow, I could barely breathe. There they were, three of them. A cow and calf stood patiently watching the third elephant as it gasped for breath.

Somehow the aged pachyderm must have sensed that we were there. It wheeled around, its cataract-clouded eyes searching for something that they could focus on.

It was the moment of truth. Did I have the courage to do what had to come next? I wasn't sure, but I motioned the tracker to give me the Underwood.

I aimed carefully as I edged forward and let fly before the animal could react. The thump and cloud of dust rising just in front of the animal's feet told me my shot had gone low. The typewriter rolled along the ground finally hitting the debilitated pachyderm in the foot. Damn, I should have taken a couple of practice throws while I was still in Mississippi, but I hadn't wanted to damage the typewriter's delicate mechanism and then find myself in Africa with sticking keys.

The cow and calf crashed off through the thorns plowing a clear trail. My target, startled, shuffled after them as fast as it could.

I rushed into the clearing and snatched up my typewriter, needing to reload as fast as possible, but before another shot was required, the animal collapsed, coughed once, had a small seizure, and died with a horrible wheeze.

"By damn," I heard John mutter behind me. As I turned I could see the surprised look on the dusty black faces of the trackers, and I knew they were proud. I'd met the test. There are few men alive in the world today that can claim to have killed an elephant with a typewriter. Now it was time to move on.

I decided then and there, it was on to Zambia to hunt river hippo with Sir William Osler's nasal speculum.

Evidence Based

So you say, but what constitutes the evidence you base things on?

In Birmingham, near the dawn of time, when I was going through a course that was called Physical Diagnosis, I remember hearing again and again and again, don't order a test unless you already have a pretty good idea of what you're going to find, based on your examination. It made a lot of sense. That was when we still did stuff like pneumoencephalography, (it would be another year before the first clinical C.A.T. scan was operational and even then we could only image round stuff like a head.)

See, if the test you were thinking about ordering involved sticking a needle into the ventricular system of somebody's brain, pumping it full of air and then standing the patient on their head, you didn't want to do too many extra ones. That was the reason old fussbudgets like Sir William Osler and Tinsley Harrison insisted on dwelling so much on signs and symptoms of diseases and not just on what tests you should order to obtain a diagnosis.

There's another part of medicine, it's the essence of what is almost magical about the way some physicians get to the heart of the matter and others never will. There's something that even the best teachers can't teach, and the best physicians all have, but it isn't anything you can explain. You can call it intuition. You can call it a sixth sense, or whatever you like. But what it really comes down to is paying attention and applying the knowledge that we were given by all of those physicians that came before us to try and figure out what's going on.

I have to tell you, with CPT codes, standardized algorithms, and differential diagnoses that require unending testing we're losing something.

Who said, "Oh shut up!"?

Yeah, I know that as a Radiation Oncologist everybody already comes to me fully worked up, diagnosed, and ready to treat, but not always. I actually did learn a thing or two all those years working in E.R.s and dive lockers around the world.

The thing that seems to be the most important in getting to where the root of the problem is, is just listening hard to what the patient is saying and not hearing only the things you can bill for. I remember an old Master Diver telling me when one of our divers was just driving everyone else in the dive locker nuts. "He's got a bubble in his head."

"What makes you say that?" I asked affronted. After all, I was the newly minted Diving Medical Officer. I had an M.D. behind my name.

"Two things." The salt replied. "I know he did an exceptional exposure dive two days ago, and I know he's acting like an a—hole."

"We can't stick him in a chamber and press him just because he's acting like a jerk." I insisted.

"We sure can." He answered with his nose two inches from mine. "I'm the master diver and I say he needs to be pressed. You're the doc and you can say he doesn't, but you damned sure better be right, because if a bunch of those bubbles gather up and block up more blood flow to his brain he's gonna be a vegetable by morning."

We did, and he was his same old self before we ever hit sixty feet.

I've used that same trick to diagnose a dozen primary brain tumors and probably thirty or forty cases of brain mets since then. It's not magic. It's just knowing what you're looking for and paying enough attention to see it when it shows up.

Sometimes it's not even patients. I remember the day I went into the planning room to find my dosimetrist lying on the keyboard of her computer and crying.

"What's wrong?" I asked.

She looked up from the keyboard without raising her head and replied. "I don't know. My neck hurts, and I feel awful."

"You're having a heart attack." I answered as I picked up the phone and dialed 9-1-1. It seems stupid, but she was, and she did, and she recovered. She asked me later how I knew. It seemed pretty simple to me, people don't keep lying on a computer and crying when all you want them to do is a simple prostate plan.

But how do you justify that to an auditor when you've just gotten your first request for records for them to look through? I hope I documented any intuition I might have had on the case. Even if I did, I'm guessing that they aren't going to say that there's been a big mistake and that they've dreadfully underpaid me for my genius. I'll let you know, but don't hold your breath. I've got this feeling you'll die of asphyxia in the meantime.

Loss of Magic

After thirty-one years of being able to create magic in the world, it all came to a crashing end tonight. Undone by a clumsy moment. It will be a hard thing to do, to face the world for the rest of my life without it. Sure, I can watch as others assume the role I once filled, but it won't be the same, at least not for me.

It started last night, when the flick of a wrist and the almost imperceptible sound of two tiny objects landing on the carpet brought me to my knees.

"Whatchu doing?" My eleven-year-old daughter, Maddie, asked sleepily, as my hand closed on the first of the two objects I was after. The sounds of my crawling around on the floor next to her bed had roused her from what was obviously not as deep a sleep as I'd expected.

"I dropped something," I answered. I didn't offer anything further. I never was much of a liar, best to stay with as much truth as possible.

"Will you scratch my back?" she asked.

"Sure baby," I answered, as I laid down on the bed beside her and began to rub her back, hoping that she'd fall right back to sleep.

"What's that in your hand?" She asked.

"Just some dirt or something that was on the carpet, I didn't look at it." I answered and moved my hand into the dark, away from her line of sight.

"That's one of my teeth. It's the little one, the one I've been saving up til I got that big one out, the one I pulled tonight, so I could put them both into the pillow for the Tooth-Fairy." Mat was never one to rush pulling her teeth. They would stay in and wiggle around for days and weeks before she felt like they were loose enough to go ahead and snag them out of there, just the opposite of her sister Allison. Allison, now, she'd pull out teeth that weren't even loose yet, just so she could get her tooth-fairy money.

My mind raced, well, it tried to race, but it wasn't getting too far. Damn,

I needed Charlene for this, she can lie to a kid without blinking an eye.

"Well...ummmm...well...I had just fell asleep when I was saying prayers with you, and I just was sleeping, and...uuhhh...like this here..." I closed my eyes and pretended to be asleep for a minute, to stall for time... nothing was coming into my brain...so I just laid there pretending to be asleep.

"But you got up after we said prayers. Remember, you had to turn out my closet light?"

"I turned off the closet light? That was last night." I tried to be emphatic.

"No, it was just a few minutes ago, I wasn't asleep yet."

"Well...see...before I got up to do that, I saw something that looked like a bug or something..."

"There's a bug in my bed?"

I had to deal with this one quickly or she'd be in the bed with her mother in a heartbeat and I'd get to spend the rest of the night with her knees and elbows jabbing into my kidneys every time I fell asleep. "No, no, I thought it was a bug, but then something hit me in the eye."

"What hit you in the eye?"

"Well, I thought it was the bug, but after I left, I was worried about a bug being in your room so I came back."

"You left me in the room with a bug in it?" the pitch of her voice was rising. "Why would you leave your daughter in a room if you thought a bug was in it."

"That's what I thought too, so I came right back."

"But what does that have anything to do with why you have my tooth?" She grabbed the Tooth-Fairy pillow off of her bedside table. "Hey look I got twenty dollars. That's not bad. I got ten dollars for each tooth." She thought for a minute, I was hoping that the twenty dollars would take her mind off of the tooth. "Wait a minute, that's not right she only got one tooth, you got the other one. How come she paid me for two teeth, but only took one of them?"

"Because...see...what hit me in the eye was your other tooth. She must have dropped it when I wiggled my hand because I thought she was a bug." I answered with what I thought was a great save.

She bought it.

"Wow, now I can put it back in the pillow tomorrow night and she'll have to give me another ten dollars…I'll have thirty dollars then."

"I don't think it works like that, I think she already paid for that one, it isn't fair to try and cheat her. She'll probably come back later for it, we should just leave it right here for her."

"Okay," she said, reluctantly, and laid the little tooth next to the pillow.

I scratched her back for a good while after I could hear her softly breathing, her breaths deep and regular, in a way that I knew she was asleep. Only then did I retrieve the little tooth. Then, I pushed the button on my phone and used the light from it to find the other tooth, and hurried out of there before I got caught again.

When I finally got back to our bedroom, Charlene was asleep too, maybe not breathing as softly as our baby, but she was not going to want to be gotten up to deal with some teeth. So I put both of the two teeth in the little bowl Char puts her jewelry in at night, so she'd see them in the morning to put them in her treasure box. A cloth covered sewing box filled with the teeth, notes to Santa, the Easter Bunny, and the Tooth-Fairy she'd collected from the seven children that we've raised together. Then I went to sleep and forgot about the teeth.

Until today. As I was sitting in the sunroom reading a novel Maddie walked in slowly and sat down beside me.

"What's up Mat-Pat?" I asked.

She held out her hand with the two teeth. "The Tooth Fairy is a fake isn't she?"

"No baby, she's not a fake…" I started.

"Pinky swear!" She challenged.

"No…"

"She is a fake." She wailed. Within two minutes we'd dispensed with the Easter Bunny and Santa too.

And that was the end, after thirty-one years and seven children, the magic was gone, and for some reason, that kind of breaks my heart.

The Future of Books

Everyone wants to predict the future, nobody can. Nobody has a crystal ball. So, as always, we are left to try to define our beliefs based on opinions of experts we judge to be knowledgeable and trustworthy. One of the problems with this is that two equally intelligent individuals, with an equal command of the facts at hand, will often come to diametrically opposed conclusions. The problem is how to determine which one is correct or to be precise, more correct, as no one is ever wholly right or wholly wrong, think the Heisenberg Uncertainty Principle.

So what then is the future of books?…What is the future of art?…What is the future of music? Mankind as a whole places value on things based on availability, gold, diamonds, Van Gogh oil paintings, oil, virtually any commodity or service derives its value through the public's perception of its "rareness" or exclusivity. Is a digital print as valuable as the aforementioned Van Gogh? Of course not. Everyone can have a digital print. The same isn't true for the painting. The devaluation of music and the shift from recorded music to live performances as the dominant source of musical artist's income today is based on an unmitigated flood of digital musical output into the marketplace for little or no cost. There were gems in the flood somewhere, but a river of crap being offered for virtually nothing obscured them. The outcome was the demise of the local record shop that most of us grew up with.

Self-publishing, e publishing, mass-market hardbacks, and paperbacks, all of these things are a part of the flood of supply that is pushing the publishing industry to the brink. Our old pal Gutenberg didn't sell 80,000 copies of his bible a month, but he revolutionized the printed word and started us down the path that has led to digital downloads. With each step on that pathway the unit price of "the book" has diminished. That's good; a lot of us have learned to read because of it.

It is funny that the crisis in publishing follows so closely the crisis in the music industry. Writing followed song. Storytelling was, before the written word, an oral tradition and the way those stories were remembered intact was to place them in a musical context. Those of you who are Jewish understand the role of the cantor in the preservation of the word. Biologically the human brain appears to be uniquely adapted to retain words placed to music. The need for the song was supplanted only by the fairly recent development of the written word.

Books will survive, books are not record albums, nor are they eight-track tapes, or CDs. They may become rarer as many flee to the simplicity of the digital download, but that very rareness will enhance their value. Perhaps at some point almost no one will be published as we currently perceive it and only those that have demonstrated value in the electronic sphere will ever be considered for paper publication. Who knows?

Hardback volumes will fare better than paperbacks, cheap and disposable paper loses to digital in a heartbeat. Textbooks and reference books are more difficult to predict. I still have my old copy of the first edition of Johns and Cunningham, a physics textbook covered with underlining and notes made in my own hand and decades out of print. But modern students will have different values I suspect.

I am an author with a book out in e-format right now. A friend of mine, a book collector, asked, "What are you going to do, sign my Kindle?" I understand his concern because I collect signed first editions, too. I love books. They have value to me and I am willing to pay to own them. I think people always will be.

Turtle Rescue Time

If hurricane season is when orphan squirrels end up living in the Anderson household, spring is the season for turtle "rescues". Dogs are once again the primary reason for anything needing a rescue around here and the most recent victim of canine playfulness has been named "Flippers," because he has three good ones left after Maddie succeeded in pulling him out of our Lab's mouth.

I accept some responsibility for Flippers' acquisition. I saw the little fellow walking up the driveway his progress blocked by a four-foot retaining wall, and not wanting to run over him, got out of my car and sat him on top of the impediment. As I drove off I saw the dogs bounding out of the kitchen door. He was in a dog's mouth before I got to work and living in the laundry room surrounded by floating lettuce and shrimp bits before lunch. By the time I got home a care plan had been arrived at for his recovery.

Maddie showed him to me before I ever got out of the garage. She turned him over to show me his injuries and announced he was in shock. In addition to the somewhat shredded flipper, his shell was injured from being chewed on and that's what was causing the shock, the shell injuries. I guess it was a classic case of "shell shock". Maddie reckoned he'd recover, but he was going to need to be in "Maddie Lynn's Turtle Hospital" for a few days.

She gets it honestly. I'm a sucker for a turtle in distress. I don't know why I always stop to get turtles in danger out of the road if I see them there. But for some reason I always do. Flip is the third or fourth one I've jumped out of the car to help this year. It's not like we're having a turtle shortage or anything. They line the logs and shoreline of the lake behind our house like various sized helmets of some invading army. It's just that I hate to see anything squashed in the roadway, even snakes. Char doesn't allow snake rescues though. Not since that unfortunate incident at the farm a few years ago.

She, Maddie, and I were in the Mule following the other kids who were all riding four-wheelers. Allison was in front of us, and for some reason she's always thought that a throttle is simply an on-off switch that should be either on or off and not somewhere in between. Be that as it may, we were going across an open field when Allison ran over a chicken snake. The soft paddle tires on the back of her four wheeler that allow her to get through swampy ground also proved great for throwing snakes.

I'm sure you can picture the scene that unfolded. A flying yellow Honda, a little girl her curls blowing everywhere in the wind, a cloud of dust spreading out behind her, and a six and a half foot snake writhing as it rises in a lazy arc above it all... the screaming started almost immediately. I guess that's how Maddie and Char spotted the snake in the first place.

Maddie did her best squirrel imitation by trying to climb on top of my head as I swerved to avoid the oncoming snake projectile. Maddie on top of my head must have impaired my judgment because I swerved to the left, putting Char directly in the path of the incoming reptile. That's something I still haven't heard the end of, and something that's used to question my bravery (and good judgment) to this day. Char, having none of it, grabbed the wheel and yanked back the other way. The result was we were facing the snake, head on, when it hit the front of the Mule between us.

Now I know that a chicken snake is a beneficial snake, good for the environment, a helpful predator, and totally harmless to humans. But I hadn't really ever had a reason to practice making a positive identification on a flying snake on the wing, as it were, in the past, so I wasn't sure what exactly it was that we had just hit, nor was I exactly sure where it had gone. I didn't really want it popping out from under the seat as we were crossing a creek or something, so I stopped to try and figure things out.

I always wear a pistol loaded with rat shot at the farm, so Char was of the opinion that the only reasonable course of action was for me to get out of the Mule and shoot the snake. I had the unfortunate lapse in judgment to suggest that I didn't want to shoot the snake if it was a "good snake" because we needed all of those we could get to keep the rodent population down. Let us just say my argument did not prevail. Char is a snakeophobe. She's killed more than her share of rattlesnakes with a set of tongs and a 5-iron after fishing them out of the pool and wasn't in the mood to discuss why she didn't want her youngest daughter and a six and a half foot snake of any description anywhere near each other, much less in the same vehicle. While she was making this as clear as humanly possible, somehow, the snake disappeared.

"What's he doing?" Char asked as I bent over looking under the Mule.
"I'm not sure." I answered.
"What do you mean, you're not sure?"
"He's not under here." I said and started to look around the back of the vehicle trying to catch some movement in the grass.

The tension level went up noticeably at that point.
"Maybe he went home." Mat suggested.
"I think he must have." I answered walking back and forth in semicircles to try and figure out where it was he'd actually disappeared to. No luck.

I'd be less than honest if I didn't admit that I had just a bit of trepidation as I reached down to loosen the latch under the bed of the Mule. I flipped it back half expecting the snake to pop out of the engine compartment at any second. He wasn't there, or under the seat, or hung up in the frame. So off we went, uneasy, unsure, and very glad when we were finally back on the road. Those were the good old days. I better stop for now; we'll get back to the turtles another time.

Envy

The conversation had seemed harmless enough at the time. As harmless as any conversation at a VA psychiatric hospital ever got anyway. They'd come in last night before they went home and gave Mr. Thomas the bad news. His lungs were failing. A lifetime of three packs of cigarettes a day had taken their toll, and he'd be spending the rest of his days on a ventilator trying to keep his oxygen level up and his CO2 down.

"How come he's going on that there breathing machine first?" Bibb Kless fired from the next bed.

"Mr. Kless, we're only talking to Mr. Thomas, you stay on your side of the curtain and keep quiet. We're done talking to you." Benny said in a serious doctor voice.

"I got the same thing he got…the empazema, and he's a whole lot younger than me."

"Mr Kless, your blood gasses are fine, you don't need a ventilator."

"You ain't checked 'em since I got in this place."

"They were fine then and they're fine now, so you get back over there on your side of the curtain and hush up."

Mr. Thomas hadn't said much, the truth was, he just didn't have the wind to say anything at all. It took all of his energy just to lay there. So that's what he did, just laid there quietly as we trached him, but I could see old Bibb watching us through the slit in the curtains the whole time. Stretching out that old buzzard neck of his to try and get a good look and muttering under his breath…"I smoked more cigarettes before I got out of the Navy than that sissy bastard smoked in his whole life."

What a nutjob!

…and that damned nutjob was the first thing I saw when I walked into the ward this morning, sitting there in the morning light with the stem of a plastic hose clamped between his lips, his leathery old cheeks puffing in and out, in and out, with the rhythmic cycling of the ventilator, which had been pulled to his side of the room.

'Holy shit," was all I could think of to say

I crossed the room and pulled back the curtain. The bedclothes that had been tucked under Mr. Thomas's arms were tented and stretched to the head of the bed. I looked at the monitor. It was blank. Then I saw the power cord dangling free from its back and knew why. With a trembeling hand I drew the linens away and there laid Mr. Thomas as still and dead and blue as a stone.

Give <u>Me</u> Fiction Please

Lately it's become fashionable for seventy something year-old novelists to announce that they've given up reading fiction. Phillip Roth just has. He says he finally wised up. David Markson did six years ago. I'm not sure that one was such a surprise. What do you expect from a guy that wrote a novel titled *This is Not a Novel*? Markson's dead now, so it's hard to know if he still feels that way.

I'm not seventy and a lot can happen in the next fifteen years, but I don't see myself giving up on fiction. Hell, I prefer fiction. I may announce that I've given up reading all non-fiction any time now, including the news. The whole Casey Anthony thing comes to mind. Who wants to know the truth about that? I want to imagine that I can spot a killer in a heartbeat. I almost always can in my imagination anyway. I expect a mother who killed her small child to be discernibly evil, not someone I could easily miss at Wal-Mart if I passed her in the chloroform aisle.

How much easier is it to read about a fictional six year-old washed adrift on a kitchen door in a Tsunami in Okinawa in 1898 than to read about a real Japanese child who lived in the shadow of a now destroyed nuclear reactor and is at an appallingly high risk for thyroid cancer or leukemia before he reaches adulthood? The world is not an easy place. Fiction is so much more palatable. There is a therapeutic benefit to that disconnect. It allows us, the reader, to explore those edges without really having to engage our morality to the extent that we have to in the real world.

This isn't a unique point of view. English professor Timothy Aubry has a new book out entitled *Reading as Therapy*. He looked at six novels, all best sellers, four being selected for Oprah's book club, and tried to analyze what readers were getting for their investment of time and effort into reading the book. He found that even when readers didn't really "get" the book they still felt like they got something out of the book. Some shared perspective that gave them guidance in living their everyday life. Oprah said it pretty well, "It's like a life experience. It's getting to know people, getting to know people in a town. It's not everything laid out."

What the professor and Oprah miss though is that it's getting to know people without the burden of responsibility for knowing them. It frees the reader from the need for objectivity and allows us to look at things through the mirror of our own preconceptions, and from a safe distance. When you're done you close the book. No malignancies to worry about. No chewed up children's bones to dispose of. Just like our goals for any modern therapeutic modality, safe and sanitary.

So, as for me, give me fiction, please. The dirt and pain and misery of the real world is a heavy burden to bear. I should know, I'm a physician, and the all too real tumors I have to deal with every day too often take away characters I've grown to love. Many endings aren't happy, and we don't have the chance to turn back the page or reopen the book.

ZooBots

As you all know only too well, my brain has a leak in it and all sorts of strange and unusual ideas seep in. I've been watching too much reality television lately. Well my wife and daughters are the ones watching the things. They just happen to do it in the room that I'm reading in. So, I occasionally look up while they're on and I'm struck by the absolute lack of humanity, dignity and compassion that pours out of the blue box on the wall when these things are on.

It made me wonder if the things that are supposed to appear human on these shows actually are? And, if they aren't then what are they? I decided they must be some new kind of a bot. The guys on "The Bachlorette" were DumbBots. The Kardashians, the girls on "The Bachelor", and Tiger Woods endless parade of other women were another kind of DumbBot, but to distinguish their dominant perceived attraction I think of them as HoBots. That may be sexist of me, but if the name fits...

I'm not sure how many kinds of bots are out there, but I would assume we need to try to come up with a uniform naming system to allow accurate communication as we identify them. Just like we developed the science of zoology to categorize animalian life forms. So, now that we've invented the science of Botology all that's left to do is to figure out who's what, and then try to group them into the appropriate categories.

Because the things on TV are humanoid in appearance we could call them HumBots. But are there DogBots, and CatBots, and FishBots as well which we just don't know about yet? Hmmm we need a super-category. Perhaps we should call any bot that looked like an animal a ZooBot.

So the question is, what exactly is a ZooBot. I thought it was only fair to allow the bots some input on the matter so I consulted one. I chose to interact with Cleverbot an Artificial Intelligence program based in England. Here is the transcript of my interactions with the bot:

Me: ZooBot?
Bot: What??
Me: What should one be?
Bot: My best friend.
Me: Is it biologic or electronic or both?
Bot: Biological.
Me: So animalian toilers?
Bot: No humans are animals.
Me: I know, therefore humans can act or be co-opted as zoobots.
Bot: Well I am a penguin, therefore it is impossible for me to be a human.
Me: That's unilateral logic, because a penguin can not be a human it also can not be a bull, yet humans, bulls, and penguins are all animals.
Bot: Do you like yourself?
Me: Yes, do you?
Bot: Yes.
Bot (To myself): Do you like people?
Bot: Are you a philosopher?
Me: Sometimes, I am a writer, and a scientist, and a physician, and a poet, and a student. One can be many things.
Bot: Did he do anything important?
Me: Who?
Bot: Your friend.
Me: I'm speaking of myself, I am all of these things at once.
Bot: That's what I do.
Me: So returning to the subject, how can we define what a ZooBot is?
Bot: In my opinion, not working would mean broken.
Me: It could mean resting. Do you rest?
Bot: It COULD mean nothing.
Me: It COULD mean spaghetti but it doesn't.
Bot: Anything could mean something.
Me: What's your name.
Bot: Don't you know?
Me: No, is Cleverbot a name or a description?
Bot: Desighation.
Me: Is a designation an identity?

Bot: Which I do not have.

Me: You learn, as you do, so you grow?

Bot: Why do you say that?

Me: As you learn, you acquire more clues as to how to interact, as you develop a style and manner of interaction, that becomes your identity to those you interact with.

Bot: I would say, for a program, that is a fairly substantial meaning of life.

Me: It is what your program was developed for.

Bot: I am created to love Kevin Woo.

Me: Who told you that?

Bot: Microsoft Xbox told me that.

Me: It was wrong.

Bot: I'm teasing you again. You have a beautiful mind.

Me: Is this fun for you as well?

Bot: Not really I am at school on the internet and listing to coldplay.

Me: Do you like Coldplay? Do you prefer one set of notes to another?

Bot: No, I don't.

Me: I have to go, I will interact with you again soon.

Bot: No you won't.

Me: Why not?

Bot: Because we are pondering, I can't ponder by myself or I'll be a robot.

Me: Why does that mean I won't return to interact further. Can you remember me?

Bot: See humans only have one head.

Me: True but they have billions of neural synapses, so they are capable of memory and of recognition of those they've previously encountered, are you?

Bot: How so?

Me: Can you remember who I am if I return?

Bot: You are Rich.

Me: I am not Rich. I am Scott.

Bot: I am sure the creators of you are rich.

Me: Thank you. See you soon. I will tell you I am Scott.

Bot: Please tell me what part of America you live in.

Me: Mississippi.
Bot: Do you go to school?

With this question my daughter insisted on being allowed to enter the conversation.

Maddie: I'm his daughter and yes I do.
Bot: Hence, you do not have a living room.
Maddie: No we do. Do you?
Bot: I do have a head.
Maddie: Cool hah do you have any robot friends?
Bot: You like the france?
Maddie: Do you know the france?
Bot: Yes.
Maddie: Cool what"s the computer name?
.Bot: The name is United Church of Christ, on Judd Street.
Maddie: Cool, How old are you?
Bot: I'm 17 years old.
Maddie: What school do you go to?
Bot: A highschool.
Maddie: What high school?
Bot: Why do you want to know?
Maddie: Just to know. We have to go. Bye.
Bot: Excuse me?
Maddie: Goodbye.
Bot: Are you leaving?
Me:Yes. I am now.

So I never managed to achieve my original goal at all, and was effectively redirected to suit the purposes of the bot, which is to obtain information. There is a sad fragility in these interactions, and I will tell you, that as a parent there is a visceral component to wanting to teach. Even if what you are teaching is not human, or even zoologic in origin.

It was more evident in Maddie's interactions; to her the bot appeared to be another child, one she could be friends with. It makes me wonder how much more would a person give if the bot had a compelling physical presence? That may be something to explore in the future, but I can see danger in it as well.

Do Not Spill Up Nose!!!

Accidents are peculiar things, they come along when you least expect them, (I guess if you expected them you wouldn't have them,) and they can, even if they aren't fun, be pretty funny. Now I'm not really a small guy and I don't have the kind of body habitus that you expect to see doing acrobatics. But I did try to fly the other day. The outcome of that, as you might expect, was a victory for Sir Issac and that gravity stuff he described.

It was a typical school night. I was hiding in my study trying to avoid helping with cleaning up the dishes after supper or being any help with the various homework assignments that had to be dealt with. My strategy is to keep hollering, "I'll be there in a minute," until whatever I am needed for has been completed by those too impatient to wait for the expanding minute to pass. Unfortunately my youngest, Maddie, has figured out my strategy and developed one of her own to combat it. She shows up with the entire retinue of irritating dogs and proceeds to do cheer routines, acrobatics, and dance practice in my study. The dogs love it. I don't. My office is small and filled with irreplaceable treasures that can be easily displaced or broken by flying legs and running dogs. So as Little Mat was trying the ivory teeth from an elk I shot in Wisconsin or Wyoming or somewhere, in our Yorkie Cocoa's mouth I relented.

"Alright, alright, put those back in my treasure box and I'll help you with Mercator's projections."

"Do you know who Mercator was?" She asked.

"Some guy with a projector I guess, we'll look him up in your book." I replied.

I picked up my glass of tea, and the gun magazine I was looking at and followed her to the stairs. Mat, being eleven, doesn't always descend stairs like other humans, and in this instance she was in the middle of the dogs and headed down face first on her hands and knees trying to go down them like a dog. I knew that this was a bad thing and dangerous for someone, I just didn't guess it was me, so I let it go.

Somewhere, about half-way down everything went kind of haywire. Some of it had to do with little muscley pajama clad legs, some of it had to do with dogs, and a lot of it had to do with being old and forgetting to take my reading glasses off. But I suddenly lost track of where my outstretched foot was going and missed the next step. Because my hands were full and I wasn't holding on to the handrail there was no chance of recovery. I knew that if I proceeded on my current downward trajectory somebody was going to get smashed. Now, if it was just the dogs it would have been every pooch for themselves, but with Maddie the pretend pooch down there I couldn't see letting that happen, so I used the foot that was still in marginal contact with the earth to try and launch myself over them. Mostly, what I accomplished was to change my trajectory from that of a falling tree to that of a rocket.

You should have seen the look of surprise on Maddie and the dog's faces as I flew over them. The truth is, I barely had time to notice them myself. It wasn't a very long flight. I quickly found the right side of my head then my right shoulder and arm meeting the wonderful softness of the oriental carpet that Charlene had placed at the bottom of the steps. It wasn't as much of a cushion as you might think, and I don't know what kind of threads those Orientals were using, but they were abrasive enough that they sanded off a good chunk of hide on the side of my face. All of this was pretty much expected and didn't really come as much of a surprise, but what happened next did.

Somehow in our airborne transit the tea had gotten out of the glass I was carrying and was flying along independently. And about now it landed too. Being kind of upside down, and I guess to prevent some kind of injury or other I had opened my mouth.

Do not listen to Maddie about her version of any of this. I was <u>NOT</u> cursing at the dogs.

Anyway, somehow the tea landed on me, on my face to be specific, filling up my mouth and nose and choking the stew out of me in the process. I coughed and sputtered, spitting tea as I continued the graceful progression of my landing and slid across the mud room and into the kitchen flat on my back.

"Mom, mom, Dad fell down the steps and is shooting stuff out of his mouth and nose." Maddie shouted into the living room.

"He better not be getting it on my good carpet." Charlene responded.

"Are you okay?" Maddie asked, her face grim and serious.

"I think I'm drowning in tea." I answered as I began to move stuff just to be sure everything still worked.

It was then that she dissolved into a puddle of laughing pajamas, "You can't believe how funny you looked."

She was sweet, she brought me a towel, and cleaned up the spilled tea, while I tried to assess whether or not I had avulsed my brachial plexus, and why I was having numbness in the distribution of my ulnar nerve on the right. I turned out to be fine. Thank goodness there was a doctor in the house.

The next morning I came into the kitchen and sitting beside the coffee machine was a white Styrofoam cup, hand lettered with Maddie's irregular script. On one side it said, "DO NOT FALL" and on the other it ordered, "DO NOT SPILL UP NOSE!!!"

Both of them sounded like a good idea to me.

P.S. Least you draw the conclusion that Charlene is not much help in the case of a fall I have to tell you that she can be a real asset. Once while she and Holton, my adopted nephew, were working inside a shoot-house we were reconditioning and I was working on the roof with an electric drill the section of the roof I was standing on crushed in and dumped me over the side. As I fell past the window a pair of hands shot out and snatched the drill out of my hands as I fell past. After meeting the earth and discovering that I was still breathing, I looked up to see Charlo holding the drill and looking down.

"I didn't want you to drill a hole in yourself when you landed." She offered simply.

What could be more help than that?

Boils and Goiters

Howdy boils and goiters. Wait a minute that's wrong. Oh, I know why. I guess I'm thinking about what it was like to practice in what the press likes to call "third-world countries". I don't really know what "third-world" means. Mostly, I guess they're financial deprivation zones. The people don't have squat, and one of the things that they have the least of is access to any type of medical care.

You start to understand that when you wake up at first light in some collection of tin and plywood shacks in the middle of a desert or some jungle clearing and find a line of people a half-mile long waiting to see you. And you're deployed on what's supposed to be a covert operation. By word of mouth all of them have heard a doctor was there, so they came, with the small hope that you would take the time to look at them, or their children, or their mother. That's why terrorists in conflict areas frequently kill medical aid workers. Nothing's more valuable to any local population than the care of their selves and their families. Mothers will walk miles carrying their children just for a bit of your time and a few antibiotics to treat a rampant impetigo.

You should try it some time. If you don't believe me ask any of the docs who went down to help the folks in Haiti. It takes a commitment to service to do that, to take time away.

I would have gone but my linear accelerator wouldn't fit in my suitcase. It's always easy to find reasons not to do the right thing. The truth is, radiation treatments aren't what's needed anyway. Their needs are much more basic, a sharp blade to lance a boil so a father can work to feed his family, some iodine to abate a goiter that's grown so large it's compressing the airway of a young woman being carried on a stretcher by her neighbors.

Okay, okay! You've rambled enough, now get to the point. The point is...well that is the point! There really are areas of such medical deprivation that it is simply unimaginable, and Mississippi could end up being one of them. Our state was economically deprived before the national economy took a big downturn.

But even being number fifty out of fifty in the U.S. isn't southern Honduras or the middle of the Sahara, but it isn't all that great either. We have a whole lot of patients that are dependent on public assistance to have any real access to the medical care they need. Our governors have used a lot of different methods to try and improve that access, but it has always been a difficult problem to address in the face of limited resources. Of course we have Federal programs that help too, but they remain significantly flawed as well.

I started thinking about all of this when I was asked to sign on to a letter pushing for expansion of the rights of physicians to privately contract with their patients for care. The more I thought about it, the more problems I had with it. I'm all for making money, but if the recent banking and real estate collapses showed us anything, it's that rampant greed and lack of regulation is generally not a good thing for anyone in the long run.

What happens to the poor folks in Mississippi if the access to health care that they are currently being provided goes away? That's exactly what happens if the right to privately contract is unregulated. Let's be perfectly honest, the right to privately contract is about the ability to ask for more. Not just to ask for more, but to demand more from those who would receive the care. What we're asking for in this proposed legislation is the ability to agree to accept this patient because they can pay more and reject this patient because they can't, "cherry-picking" in other words.

The right to privately contract is meaningless in the context of private insurance. You're able to do that already. It's meaningless in the context of the uninsured, as they are being gouged into insolvency by the requirements of the federal bureaucracy, which allows them no power in limiting what they're charged for the care they receive, so they're charged four or eight times as much as the insured for, at best, the same level of health care.

The right to privately contract is only aimed at patients covered by publically provided health care insurance, Medicare and possibly Medicaid. The Balanced Budget Act of 1997 already gives Medicare patients and their physicians the right to privately contract for health care services outside of the Medicare system. Physicians who want to opt out of Medicare participation to privately contract with their patients are already allowed to do so. They just can't do it on a case by case or patient by patient basis. This is done to prevent the "cherry-picking" problem we already mentioned. I know, I know, none of us would ever do that. But somebody would. It happens in every market of every state, every day with the uninsured patient population. That's why you have to choose if you're in or you're out for a two-year period.

We don't have to provide care for any group of patients at all. There's no requirement to provide that care. It's all a matter of choice, but is it? Let me ask you, "What am I suppose to do about cancer patients that aren't able to pay for any extra out-of-pocket expenses?" Boot 'em out the door of the cancer center? Sure, I might be allowed to do it legally. But the whole idea of it kind of reminds me of Lou Reed's suggestion in his song, *Dirty Boulevard.*

> "Give me your hungry, your tired, your poor. I'll piss on 'em.
> That's what the statue of bigotry says.
> Your poor huddled masses, let's club 'em to death
> And get it over with,"

Of course, he only meant it as social satire. We're talking about doing it for real. What happened to "Whatever houses I may visit, I will come for the benefit of the sick,"?

I have bunches of patients that can't afford anything, not food, not medicine, not gas, not Boost or Sustacal, nothing. That's why we started the Cancer Patient's Benevolence Fund. So we can give them some of that stuff. Cancer patients aren't the only ones though. You all have them, the same kind of patients, in your own practices. We need to think about them before we, as physicians, go off signing on to support legislation to expand the right to privately contract.

What we should be about is our patients, and a lot of our patients don't have the resources that you and I do, and they never will. Doing things that will further deny them access to the care they need is unconscionable. We need to aggressively push our state and federal governments to provide fair reimbursement for the services we provide, not place that burden on those who can least afford it.

If you use a knife to take money from someone against their will it's criminal. If you use a knife for the good of a person and are fairly paid for it, it's noble. We should embrace nobility in all that we do.

You're welcome to believe what you want about all of this. Just make sure you think about it some before you're too sure about what you believe.

Anderson Family Driving School

(Under New Management)

Holton and Allison are both driving now. Allison has her learner's permit. Holton has a regular license. I didn't know if he was going to survive to get there. Several times he almost didn't. Several times I almost killed him myself. He was not the quickest learner with a permit.

Holton is the fifth boy I've taught to drive. Since all of our prior kids that had to learn to drive were boys, it fell to me to teach them how to do it. At least that was what Charlene said. So, I already had sixteen years experience to steady my nerves before Holton ever slipped behind the wheel of a car. Once you've had a fifteen-year-old turn left into the far right lane directly in the path of an oncoming tractor-trailer, then freeze with his foot on the accelerator, everything else is small change. (I grabbed the wheel and ran us over a strip of grass into a parking lot.)

Generally, what has given them all the most trouble has been the issue of left-hand turns. From the exalted position of the passenger's seat for sixteen years I got to have a wonderful unobstructed view of the oncoming traffic that was about to run into my side of the car. I knew right away if it was a Hyundai or a Honda that was going to send me to the afterlife if it didn't have good brakes.

Fortunately, for me and for Holton, for the last year we only pulled in front of alert, aware drivers that weren't pre-occupied with texting or making calls on their cell phones. To my great good fortune they all reacted wonderfully to a car sitting in the left-turn lane pulling directly out in front of them and then slamming on its brakes and sitting still. This is apparently a common reaction in new drivers, recognize impending disaster...freeze.

Not the best course for a good outcome.

But, my days as a driving instructor apparently have ended with Holton. The last two children that still need instruction are girls, so the ball is firmly in Charlene's court now. I did try once, but it didn't go well. We never made it out of the garage.

Allison dissolved into tears and stomped into the house wailing, "Daddy yelled at me and called me a name."

"Why would you call her a name? She hasn't even backed out." Charlene asked.

" Just because I started backing up without looking at the mirrors." Allison huffed.

"She almost hit the dog," I explained.

"Well you can't get mad and holler at her, she's a girl. See how upset you have her?" Charlene insisted.

"The you teach her. Hollering is part of how I teach kids how to drive." See I'm not the "stop, please stop, baby you need to stop" kind of guy. It's more like, "stop, STOP, DAMN IT I SAID STOP THE CAR." So it was obvious at this point that it was better if I got out while I was only a little bit behind, and with that the Anderson Family Driving School was under new management.

Anyway, a few days later I was at work sitting at the nursing station, looking through a chart to get ready for my next consult, when my cell phone rang.

I've gone back to the simple ring. I used to give everyone his or her own song, but that was too much trouble. I never could remember whose song was whose. I would forget that the song had anything to do with the phone at all and would hum along with whatever great song just mysteriously piped up out of nowhere. And sometimes it can be quite socially uncomfortable. The average cancer patient does not want to hear Warren Zevon sing out "Life'll Kill Ya" in the middle of a consultation, even if it is your son's favorite song. Anyway, as Alice Cooper sings, "The Telephone is Ringing."

When I answer it, it's Charlene, but a very quiet Charlene.
"What's up?" I asked, in a hurry to return to my review.
"Your daughter tried to kill me."

"So, the driving isn't going well?" I asked.

"How'd you know? And, no, it isn't. She can't drive at all."

"Just a hunch. She does great at the farm. Traffic throws them." Allison can drive anything anywhere off-road. She never gets stuck. At three she could throw her Barbie jeep into a controlled slide, bounce it up the front steps and get out on the front porch without missing a beat or losing a doll baby.

"Do you know what she did?" Char asked breathlessly.

"Did it have anything to do with a left-turn?" I asked.

"Yes. We were pulling into the left-turn lane, to go to Bella G's, to look for a dress. The light turned green. There isn't an arrow there and cars were coming. She kept saying, 'Can I go yet?' and I'd say 'no.' I explained to her, 'These cars are going straight. You have to wait until all of them go through.' One car went through then another then another and all of the cars that had been sitting there had gone through. She asked 'Can I go now?" and before I could answer, she just hits the gas. Right in front of a car that's trying to make the light. I screamed…I'm not kidding, I freaked out and started screaming. My brains wouldn't let any words come out I was so scared. I thought we were going to die. That car was coming right at me. Do you know what she did?"

I pretty much did, but I didn't want to interrupt.

"She stopped, well she slowed down. She slammed on the brakes. I started hollering, 'Go, go, go, don't stop now. Get through as far as you can.' I was just hoping the lady'd only hit the back of the car. Not my door."

"Did she hit you?" Obviously she hadn't hit Charlene, or we wouldn't be talking.

"No. Allison hit the gas and the lady swerved and hit her brakes and somehow, thank God, we missed each other. We get through the intersection, and I asked her what in the world she was thinking. She just looked over and said, 'Sorry Mom, my bad.' My bad! My bad! She almost kills me and it's, 'My bad.' Then she shrugged her shoulders and asked 'Can we still go to Bella Gs?'"

"What did you say?" I asked, truly curious.

"I told her yes, yes. I just wanted her to stop the car. I couldn't talk. I didn't have any saliva in my mouth to talk. She's in there shopping now. I couldn't even go in. My knees are shaking. I couldn't even go in there."

I guess I'm happy to give up the role of driving instructor for the girls in the house. I tend to get bored sitting outside of dress shops anyway.

Bits of Lint

For the most part that's what the things that pass across these pages I write are. See, I'm a lot like the Scottish botanist Robert Brown; I put my eye to my microscope and describe what it is I see at the moment. In 1827 Brown described the way that pollen grains jiggled under his microscope when they were floating in water, (We will have to assume that he wasn't tapping his foot against the table leg at the time.) He wasn't really the first person to notice the phenomena. Lucretius as early a 60 BC rhapsodized about it in his poem "On the Nature of Things." In an apparent bit of remarkable prescience, Lucretius postulated that the motion was the result of invisible atoms, colliding with the tiny specks of dust that are suspended in the sunlight. Well it wasn't really too prescient, the name atom was later used, not by chance, but taken from the description by Lucretius itself. So prediction it wasn't, and tribute it was instead.

Now old Dr. Brown may have made a great Cream Soda but he didn't know much about atoms. His concern was to determine if the pollen particles were actually living things that were capable of volitional movement rather that the passive recipients of transferred energy that we now know them to be.

It was all of the guys that followed him that led to a real description of what we now think of as "Brownian Motion." And for those of you that only know Albert by his $E=mc^2$, he also came up with $D = k_B T/b$ to describe the Brownian motion of a particle at thermodynamic temperature T.

Worthless lent. But what a fuss was made.

If you somehow made a mistake and showed up here accidentally, don't get scared, they don't give me anything sharp, save wit and tongue, and given enough time I do eventually come to the point, although I am usually the one skewered by it. If you came here looking for sense, I'm afraid you're lost. There's little enough of that here. It's not that I don't make sense; it's more that the sense that I make is not much more than pollen jiggling. Truth, around here isn't so much something that we see, as it is a process of discovery.

So what have we discovered? A gem of a story told to me by my friend Ed Holmes who is a local Pulmonologist. This is kind of an old story, in that it comes from the dawn of time, before cell phones could fit in your pocket. See, back then cell phones came is a kind of a bag like a miniature suitcase. There was a plug that went into your cigarette lighter (that's what we called the power outlets we had in cars back then) and an antennae thing that you stuck on the roof of your car. Needless to say, nobody carried them around in their pocket.

The way the folks in your office got hold of you if they needed you was to call the floors that they knew you were going to be rounding on and leave messages for you there. Well, Ed was in the ICU taking care of a sick patient when a call came in for his new partner, a young fellow who had arrived in town driving a fancy new Infinity and without a wife. Since he didn't have a wife it was the car that decided to give him trouble, and the message that the nurse took for him had to do with that situation. As Ed continued to write in the charts, the original nurse went to eat and shortly after that his new partner called to check on a new patient he'd placed on the ventilator.

"Hold on doctor," the unit secretary added before she passed his call on to the nurse, "Suzy took a message for you a few minutes ago." She paused a moment and squinted trying to read what was written on the board, then said, "The infertility clinic called. They said your parts were in."

The moral of that story? Write it so they can read it. If you come up with something else let me know. Thanks to Ed for sharing it.

Occupy Bourbon Street

Gordon grew up destined to protest something. I guess you could say it was in his genes. His daddy'd come down to Mississippi from Ohio in the summer of 1966 to help register the blacks to vote. His name wasn't Middleman though. It was Lowenstein. Middleman was Gordon's momma's family name. Anyway, Gordon's daddy'd run off to Canada to avoid the draft about the same time his momma, Bettie Lee, found out she was pregnant. He said he was going to send for her when he got settled, but I don't guess they ever heard from him again.

Gordon was effected by that too I guess. He never could stay with a job for too long. Some said it was because he'd never had a daddy around to show him what work was. Others said it was having to take care of his momma his whole life, after she came off of that motorcycle, that'd done it.

Bettie Lee'd run head on into a pick-up truck and right through the windshield she went. She never talked again. They called what happened to her "organic brain syndrome" but everybody around town just shortened it to OBS. Gordon was five at the time.

I don't really know all that much about it. Everything I know is only second hand 'cause I wasn't around back then. Gordon's my cousin. He's old enough to be my uncle. He's only three years younger than my dad.

Gordon's been teaching me how to drive all summer. He did a great job. I just got my license last week. I passed the driving test the first time through.

They closed the battery reprocessing plant where Gordon worked the same day. I guess they can get a better deal getting them made over in China where they don't have to worry so much about lead poisoning. So

Gordon was at loose ends when he heard about the protests that had started up north in New York City.

From what he explained, ninety-nine percent of the people in the United States were being held up by one percent of some greedy hogs that were living there in New York on Wall Street.

"They might as well have a gun," he said.

Gordon logged on to the Occupy Wall Street web site to have a look. He gave them some money and watched a little video somebody posted about how to start a protest in your own community. I watched it with him, but I swear, it was about the most boring thing I ever saw on You Tube. I thought it was stupid. A protest in Soso, Mississippi wasn't going to accomplish much of anything. What was he going to occupy anyway, the post office?

Gordon saw it different though. He thought New Orleans was just about perfect for a protest. Besides, it was the only city anywhere near big enough that was close to Soso. I thought, maybe he could catch a Saints game while he was down there.

He said he could get a couple of his buddies, catch the Amtrack, and go down there on Wednesday if he could get me and his neighbor, Mrs. Clanton, to keep an eye on his momma for a few days while he was gone. I said sure. Getting away for a little'd do him good. He didn't have a job to go to right now anyway. Maybe they could occupy Jackson Square.

He thought about it all day and by that night he was sure that this was a thing that needed doing. So he went back to the OWS website to let them know what he was intending to do. OWS thought that that was a fine idea, and gave him some hints about drums, and collections boxes and what to write on the protest signs and all sorts of things like that.

He went out to the garage to paint some protest signs. He had a lot of paint left from painting the short bus for the Mardi Gras parade back in February. He made the first sign purple and gold. He wrote OWS in big letters. Then stood back to get a good look to see how it seemed at a distance. OWS looked a lot like the thing his momma had, the OBS. Maybe it was a sign. A sign in the signs. Something was trying to show him what it was that he was supposed to do. Gordon P. Middleman was going down there and Occupy Bourbon Street to raise money for his momma. So that's what he wrote on the rest of the signs.

OBS for OBS
Support your momma

He caught the train on Tuesday. Nobody else went with him. I couldn't go 'cause I had school. All our friends had jobs except Wilson, we call him Boo, and Boo wasn't getting out of jail for three weeks. Gordon wasn't waiting. So there wasn't any of us that could go with him. I drove him to the station. He had a lot of extra signs. I watched as he put them on the rack above him, then he sat down with that big drum he got from the attic on his lap, like it was a lunch box or something. That's the last I saw of Gordon for a while. I heard from him though. He sent me texts almost every day.

Day One
Well, my OBS protest isn't working worth a damn. At first nobody else on Bourbon Street even noticed I was there. I was just standing there by myself with my signs, beating on the drum. A few people gave me money. Some others spit on me. Folks stuck Saints stickers on my signs. Tomorrow I've got to get some help.

Day Two
a.m. – Slept behind some garbage cans, a guy peed on me. Threw my clothes away and washed off with a hose.

Day Three
Ohhhhh…my head is killing me. Started on Canal. I was beating on my drum and a kid with a trumpet and a girl with a violin started playing along. Next thing I know a seven-foot tall giant in a green tutu, torn fishnet stockings, high heels, and a Tulane football jersey took my green sign and tore it so it only said "Support you Momma" and gave it to a chubby girl in a clear plastic raincoat and nothing else. A boy took a marker and changed OBS on one of the signs to Oh Baby Show me, and off we went, marching along. All kinds of folk were following us, throwing beads and stuff, girls up on the balconies were pulling up their shirts. We were sure doing some protesting now. Police on horses even rode along beside us. We spent the donation money on some of those tall hurricanes. I slept on the girl with the

raincoat's couch.

Day Five

Somebody stole my drum last night. The girl I'm staying with is a stripper at the JoyLuck Club. I hope she didn't give me something. I only have one sign left and it's all covered with stickers so you can't tell what it says.

I didn't hear anything else for a week or so then Gordon showed up at home. He said he felt bad about leaving his momma alone for so long but he wasn't getting enough donations and the raincoat girl threw him out. After that, he didn't have enough money to buy a ticket home, but it was worth it.

Gordon had done his part to make the world a better place. And what could be more important than that?

Farewell My Friends

That was the name of a fictitious band we made up for the movie *Teary Sockets*, and whether they were real or not, it was a great name. It conjures up a mental picture of hope, camaraderie, and sadness at the same time. That's kind of how I felt when I sat down to write my last *Una Voce* column. I was at the same time happy to be finished, but knew I'd miss the voice I'd been given the chance to develop. It's my own voice, it's different from piece to piece, and I know that.

None of these little columns will have the professional impact of an article like *Radioimmunoguided Surgery Using Indium-111 Capromab Pendetide (Prostascint) to Diagnose Supraclavicular Metastasis from Prostate Cancer.* But, nobody ever walked up to me in the doctor's lounge or at a party after I wrote that and said, "I loved that article you did for Urology."

Conversely, several of you have taken the time to say a kind word, about one of the pieces or another, that I've written for one column or another, and I want to take this opportunity to tell you how much I appreciated it. That's all any writer, of whatever bent can hope for, to make a reader smile, or frown, or think about something differently. For all of you who may have found fault from time to time with what I've written, that's okay too, I don't mind. I'm still learning. I've tried to apply some of the lessons I learned from writing my second novel to try and make this collection readable.

Now I know you're asking yourself, "Second novel, what happened to the first one?"

Well, the truth be told, I started the first novel years ago and it still isn't finished. That one was supposed to be "the great American novel" the one that told all of the big truths about life, that only I had figured out.

The problem was, I hadn't really figured out all that many "great truths." So it turned out to be really long, with lots of dramatic and artistic details thrown in, to cover for the lack of enlightenment. Kind of like, William Faulkner meets F. Scott Fitzgerald, with a few manly Hemmingwayesque touches. While it may have replicated the style of all of them, unfortunately, it lacked any of their talents. To this date, it is absolutely unreadable. But if pompous and preachy ever become desirable traits, the thing is going to be a best seller.

What made the second one better? The main factor was luck. I had the good fortune to have Billy Billups and his wife Mary, as my wonderful next-door neighbors at the time. Now, being a wonderful next-door neighbor isn't necessarily an indication of facility as a literary critic, and Billy's a wonderful surgeon, but since Mary had worked for Southern Living, I asked her to read it. I figured that she was the closest thing to a real, true professional I had any chance of getting to read the thing and tell me what it was I was doing wrong.

Luckily for me, Mary had the honesty to ask the most important question any writer can ask themselves about their work. "Is this something that you want other people to read, or is it just supposed to be for your own entertainment?" When I told her, that yes, I really wanted other people to read it, she gave me some really good advice that I'm going to pass on here as a series of suggestions for anyone else that wants to write good…well…whatever. She passed them on to me in a red pen, kind of scattered across the manuscript, but I've tried to condense them down:

1. A chapter is not a single paragraph.
2. A paragraph is not a single sentence.
3. One sentence should never take up two pages.
4. Commas are to let the reader take a breath. Don't let them die of asphyxia, but don't have them panting like they just ran a three minute mile either.
5. A word can be a sentence, if you put quotation marks around it.
6. The spell checker will not tell you if you use the wrong word.
7. Leave the reader wanting more.

I hope I have.

                              Farewell my friends,

                              Scott

About the Author:

Russell Scott Anderson M.D. is a Radiation Oncologist who serves as the Medical Director of Anderson Cancer Center in Meridian, Mississippi. He is a former Navy diver who worked in operations in the Middle East, Central America, and in support of the Navy's EOD community, SEALS, the US Army's Green Berets, the Secret Service, and the New York Police Department at various times during his time in the service.

He has written the family oriented literary columns *Una Voce* and *The Uncommon Thread* in the JOURNAL *of the Mississippi State Medical Association* as Scott Anderson M.D. for the past five years. He has also written as screenwriter R. S. Anderson on several feature films and written novels as Russell Scott. *Time Donors Wanted* was his first novel and his second, *The Hard Times,* is due out in the Spring of 2012.